PEDIATRICS - LABORATORY AND CLINICAL RESEARCH

PEDIATRIC URINARY BLADDER TISSUE ENGINEERING

PEDIATRICS - LABORATORY AND CLINICAL RESEARCH

Additional books in this series can be found on Nova's website under the Series tab.

Additional e-books in this series can be found on Nova's website under the e-books tab.

CELL BIOLOGY RESEARCH PROGRESS

Additional books in this series can be found on Nova's website under the Series tab.

Additional e-books in this series can be found on Nova's website under the e-books tab.

PEDIATRICS - LABORATORY AND CLINICAL RESEARCH

PEDIATRIC URINARY BLADDER TISSUE ENGINEERING

ARUN K. SHARMA
AND
EARL Y. CHENG

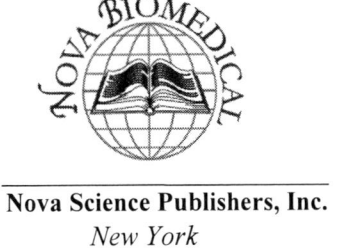

Nova Science Publishers, Inc.
New York

Copyright © 2012 by Nova Science Publishers, Inc.

All rights reserved. No part of this book may be reproduced, stored in a retrieval system or transmitted in any form or by any means: electronic, electrostatic, magnetic, tape, mechanical photocopying, recording or otherwise without the written permission of the Publisher.

For permission to use material from this book please contact us:
Telephone 631-231-7269; Fax 631-231-8175
Web Site: http://www.novapublishers.com

NOTICE TO THE READER

The Publisher has taken reasonable care in the preparation of this book, but makes no expressed or implied warranty of any kind and assumes no responsibility for any errors or omissions. No liability is assumed for incidental or consequential damages in connection with or arising out of information contained in this book. The Publisher shall not be liable for any special, consequential, or exemplary damages resulting, in whole or in part, from the readers' use of, or reliance upon, this material. Any parts of this book based on government reports are so indicated and copyright is claimed for those parts to the extent applicable to compilations of such works.

Independent verification should be sought for any data, advice or recommendations contained in this book. In addition, no responsibility is assumed by the publisher for any injury and/or damage to persons or property arising from any methods, products, instructions, ideas or otherwise contained in this publication.

This publication is designed to provide accurate and authoritative information with regard to the subject matter covered herein. It is sold with the clear understanding that the Publisher is not engaged in rendering legal or any other professional services. If legal or any other expert assistance is required, the services of a competent person should be sought. FROM A DECLARATION OF PARTICIPANTS JOINTLY ADOPTED BY A COMMITTEE OF THE AMERICAN BAR ASSOCIATION AND A COMMITTEE OF PUBLISHERS.

Additional color graphics may be available in the e-book version of this book.

Library of Congress Cataloging-in-Publication Data

Pediatric urinary bladder tissue engineering / editors, Arun K. Sharma and Earl Y. Cheng.
  p. cm.
  Includes bibliographical references and index.
  ISBN 978-1-61209-624-7 (softcover)
  1. Pediatric urology. 2. Neurogenic bladder--Treatment. 3. Tissue engineering.
I. Sharma, Arun K. II. Cheng, Earl Y.
  RJ470.P43 2011
  618.92'6--dc23
                                                                          2011031637

Published by Nova Science Publishers, Inc. † New York

Contents

Preface		vii
Chapter I	Normal Bladder Anatomy and Physiology	1
Chapter II	Etiology of the Neurogenic Bladder	3
Chapter III	Current Treatment Modalities for the Neurogenic Bladder Are Inadequate	5
Chapter IV	Advances in Tissue Engineering for Bladder Regeneration	7
Chapter V	Alternate Cell Sources for Bladder Tissue Engineering	9
Chapter VI	Bone Marrow Microenvironment	11
Chapter VII	MSC Multipotentiality and Growth Characteristics	13
Chapter VIII	The Use of MSCs as a Tool for Regenerative Medicine	15
Chapter IX	Bone Marrow Cells and Bladder Regeneration	17
Chapter X	Endothelial Progenitor Cells for Vascular Growth	19
Chapter XI	Neural Progenitor/Stem Cells	21

Chapter XII	Embryonic Stem Cells	**23**
Chapter XIII	Induced Pluripotent Stem Cells	**27**
Chapter XIV	Scaffold Material Selection: Biologics vs. Synthetics/Polymerics	**29**
Chapter XV	Controlled Delivery of Growth Factors from Scaffolds Enhances Tissue Regeneration	**33**
Chapter XVI	The Use of Nanotechnology with Self-Assembling Matrices Provides an Alternative Method of Growth Factor Delivery	**35**
Chapter XVII	Self-Asembling Nanomolecules	**37**
Chapter XVIII	PA Molecules for Tethered Growth Factor Delivery	**39**
Chapter XIX	Differentiation of Neural Progenitor Cells with IKVAV Presenting Nanofibers	**41**
Chapter XX	Summary	**43**
References		**45**
Index		**61**

Preface

Tissue engineering is a multi-disciplinary field that is continually evolving and functions through the amalgamation of principles and practices derived from materials science, clinical medicine, and the basic biological sciences. The goals of tissue engineering based therapies are to reconstitute the anatomic milieu and physiological function of diseased or damaged tissue in order to improve the poorly functioning target organ with the ultimate end goal to preserve the overall well being of the patient. With the advent of new synthetic polymers and advancements in stem cell biology, the combinatorial and/or synergistic effects of these disciplines has greatly advanced tissue engineering as a whole, particularly in the field of bladder tissue engineering.

Bladder insufficiency caused by trauma or disease including developmental defects are diagnosed each year within the United States.[1] Typical treatment options often include surgery in the form of transurethral resection; segmental or radical cystectomy; or urinary diversion in the case of bladder cancer or enterocystoplasty for those suffering from spina bifida induced neurogenic bladder.[2,3] Although these are only a few examples that illustrate the more common bladder abnormalities seen by adult and pediatric urologists alike, each of these cases demonstrate suboptimal bladder function due to aberrant cellular behavior and must be restored. Recent clinical bladder tissue engineering studies utilizing autologous cell sources of bladder cells combined with well characterized matrices led to partial restoration of bladder function of patients suffering from myelomeningocele (spina bifida).[4] Although novel in approach, the clinical outcomes of these studies displayed marginal increases in overall bladder function.

There is still a clinical need to explore novel biodegradable matrices that can be utilized in conjunction with sources of non-diseased cells that are suitable for bladder regenerative studies. This chapter will focus on the current state of bladder tissue engineering with a specific emphasis on the use of autologous and allogenic cell sources as well as biologic and synthetic matrices that influence cell growth and differentiation that can be used for future bladder tissue engineering applications.

Chapter I

Normal Bladder Anatomy and Physiology

The urinary bladder is a hollow, musculomembranous vesicle located within in the pelvic cavity that acts as a reservoir for the temporary storage and ultimate expulsion of urine through a series of highly coordinated physiological events. [5] The bladder is grossly comprised of the trigone which is the triangle shaped base of the bladder comprised of two ureteral orifices and the internal urethral orifice. The ureteral orifices provide a drainage point for urine that has been delivered by the ureters from the kidneys. The urethral orifice is the initial point of urine expulsion from the body and it should be noted that there are several distinctions between the human male and female urethra with regards to anatomy. [6, 7] Several tissue layers form the luminal and extra-luminal aspects of the bladders. The innermost portion of the bladder is comprised of the mucosa which consists of the urothelium and lamina propria. Urothelial cells line the lumen of the bladder to help create a water tight barrier between the bladder lumen and the remainder of the bladder wall through the non-exclusive expression of transmembrane and tight junction proteins. [8] Distal to the urothelium is the lamina propria which is a layer of connective tissue interspersed with blood vessels followed by the muscularis, which is also known as the detrusor muscle. The muscle component of the bladder is composed of fibers of smooth muscle cells originating from the posterior surface of the body of the pubis and runs in longitudinal directions across the internal bladder surface to the apex of the bladder and subsequently along the fundus of the bladder with intersecting fiber patterns on either side of the bladder. [9, 10] These fibers eventually insert in the prostate of the male and the vagina in females.

The function of the detrusor muscle is to aid in the rhythmic contractions for the expulsion of urine. Lastly, the outer portion of the bladder is lined with the adventitia that is almost wholly composed of connective tissue. Proper anatomical and structural arrangements of the bladder are pivotal for proper physiological function.

The contractile system of the bladder is analogous to an orchestra with many individual performers that must execute precisely as a single unit as to not create a state of discordant tones. The bladder is controlled by the autonomic nervous system with postganglionic parasympathetic neurons innervating the detrusor muscle, trigone and sphincter of the bladder. Neural control of the bladder can further be broken down into two distinct phases which include bladder storage and voiding or micturition. [11] The filling process is controlled by several mechanisms governed by somatic and sympathetic innervations. As the bladder fills, detrusor muscle activity is inhibited by sympathetic innervation as is the contractile response of the smooth muscle sphincter. Simultaneous contraction of the striated sphincter also occurs which is controlled by somatic innervation. [11-13] The process of micturition is facilitated by the relaxation of the striated sphincter, the smooth muscle sphincter and the opening of the bladder neck by somatic and sympathetic innervations while the detrusor muscle contraction is engaged by parasympathetic innervation. [11,14,15] This basic description of bladder function is typically altered in patients with a neurogenic bladder.

Chapter II

Etiology of the Neurogenic Bladder

The fundamental function of the human bladder is to provide a capacious storage reservoir that is able to store urine under low pressure and to empty to completion under volitional control. When developmental defects occur as in the case of spina bifida, a neurogenic bladder can develop resulting in loss of bladder compliance, decreased storage capacity, and/or incomplete emptying. [16] Clinical manifestations of the neurogenic bladder can include urinary incontinence, urinary tract infections, renal and bladder calculi, upper urinary tract dilatation (hydronephrosis), renal deterioration, and eventual renal failure. [17,18] As patients with a neurogenic bladder develop progressive hydronephrosis, renal injury, intractable urinary incontinence, or diminished functional capacity of the bladder due to muscle and matrix abnormalities within the bladder wall, surgical intervention is often needed. The spectrum of detrusor dysfunction in the neurogenic bladder includes areflexia, hyperreflexia, noncompliance, and detrusor-sphincter dyssynergia. [16,17,19-22] Currently, augmentation cystoplasty is the best available treatment for the end-stage neurogenic bladder. [23-26] This is accomplished by placing a detubularized segment of intestine onto the neurogenic bladder. Although functional, the incorporation of a bowel segment into the urinary tract for urinary reconstruction may lead to significant complications including infection, electrolyte abnormalities, mucus formation, stone formation, spontaneous perforation, and malignant tumor formation. [27,28] The clinical problems faced by patients with a neurogenic bladder translate into millions of dollars in health care costs.

It is estimated that the lifetime financial loss associated with the typical spina bifida patient is approximately $1 million to cover costs that include medical care, special education, and loss of income. The total societal cost of spina bifida is estimated to exceed $750 million per year, with $82 million dollars a year being paid by Social Security Administration to individuals with spina bifida. [29] Millions of dollars are also spent on medical care typically paid for by the Medicaid and Medicare Programs. Aside from the financial constraints, the emotional stress and the dramatically altered quality of life further contribute to the overall deterioration of this patient population. Therefore, measures must be taken to reduce at least a portion of the personal and societal burdens for those suffering from neurogenic bladder as consequence of developmental disease.

Chapter III

Current Treatment Modalities for the Neurogenic Bladder Are Inadequate

The aforementioned limitations of current treatment modalities have ignited the field of tissue engineering research in the hopes that bladder regeneration can become possible. Two distinctive strategies have been developed in the pursuit of bladder regeneration. The first strategy, "unseeded technology", relies upon the ingrowth of native cells to regenerate the bladder onto an implanted biodegradable scaffold. [23] Most of the research involving unseeded technology has centered on the use of small intestinal submucosa (SIS). [30] Unfortunately, unseeded technology has been hindered by scaffold contraction, variable degrees of regeneration, and a limited surface area of regenerated tissue which may be due to lack of vascularity and/or variability in the scaffold material itself. The second strategy for bladder regeneration involves "seeded technology." [30-32] Recent studies specific to the bladder have shown that seeded technology may offer significant advantages over unseeded technology. Bladder regeneration is accomplished with this technique by first obtaining bladder tissue via open or endoscopic biopsy and establishing primary bladder smooth muscle cells and urothelial cells cultures in the laboratory. The cells are then expanded ex vivo and seeded on a biodegradable membrane, which can either be synthetic or biologic polymers such as poly(glycolic acid) (PGA) and poly(1,8-octanediol-citrate) (POC) or SIS, respectively. The cell-scaffold composite graft is then re-implanted into the host where further bladder regeneration can occur.

The seeded technique has been successfully demonstrated in a number of animal models. [26,31, 33] Regenerated bladder tissue has been found histologically to be similar to normal bladder tissue with complete development of all three layers of the normal bladder (urothelium, smooth muscle, and serosa) and infiltration of well-formed blood vessels.

Chapter IV

Advances in Tissue Engineering for Bladder Regeneration

New data gathered from successful bladder regenerative studies in animals has led to a preliminary clinical trial utilizing autologous sources of bladder cells. Atala et al have demonstrated the use of non-coated synthetic scaffolds in a bladder regenerative setting. [4] Autologous sources of neurogenic urothelial and smooth muscle cells derived from myelo meningocele patients were isolated and expanded ex vivo and then seeded upon collagen or collagen/PGA scaffold composites. Subsequent re-implantation studies with a mean 46 month follow-up utilizing only collagen scaffolds resulted in no statistically significant improvement in a variety of urodynamic functions while other scaffold combinations showed a modest increase in bladder capacity. Although novel in approach, this study fails to address the possibility that the use of neurogenic bladder cells may eventually result in the reformation of a diseased bladder state over time as well as the decline in urodynamic function of patients receiving this treatment. Thus, there is great concern that the use of pathologically abnormal neurogenic cells will not result in regenerated tissue that is normal in composition and function. Extensive characterization of bladder derived neurogenic cells from our lab indicates that cultured neurogenic bladder smooth muscle cells possess and maintain different characteristics than normal smooth muscle cells in vitro. [34, 35] Further characterization of these cells demonstrate a constitutive over-expression of bFGF causes an increase in smooth muscle cell proliferation which may result in reduced bladder contractiliy. [35].

In addition, the bladders that have been augmented with autologous bladder cell sources continue to be non-contractile requiring patients to be maintained on intermittent catheterization which may in part be related to the neurogenic origin of the seeded cells. These results have further caused concern that the use of neurogenic bladder cells in seeded techniques to promote bladder regeneration may be inappropriate and an alternative cell source should be sought.

Chapter V

Alternate Cell Sources for Bladder Tissue Engineering

In order to recapitulate a physiologically functional bladder environment for tissue engineering purposes, specific cells need to be harvested and manipulated that can either mimic bladder cell function or transdifferentiate into the various components of the bladder wall including smooth muscle cells, urothelial cells, nerve cells, and a vasculature supply capable of providing adequate nutrients to the regenerating tissue. These cells are derived from sources that encompass a wide assortment of tissues including bone marrow (mesenchymal and endothelial progenitor cells); embryological tissue (embryonic stem cells), terminally differentiated dermal fibroblasts (induced pluripotent stem cells) and neural derived tissue (neural progenitor and stem cells). The multipotent attributes of these cells are exceptional sources for the regenerative process. We will explore the characteristics of each of these cell types and there use in bladder regeneration.

Chapter VI

The Bone Marrow Microenvironment

Typical human long bones contain a vast array of marrow containing elements and are organized into vascular and hematopoietic compartments comprising three main cellular systems that are found within the bone marrow cavity. These include cells of hematopoietic, endothelial, and stromal origin. [36-38] Bone marrow provides mature blood cells derived from undifferentiated stem and progenitor cells in a complex cascade of maturational and divisional steps. The bone marrow cavity is also lined with stroma at the marrow/periosteum interface in which hematopoietic and non-hematopoietic stem cells reside and receive microenvironmental cues for mobilization and differentiation. Hematopoietic stroma physically supports the differentiation of primitive hematopoietic stem cells (HSCs) that is comprised of a hierarchy of cells that have the ability to either self-renew or terminally differentiate into daughter cells with more specified functions. [39-42] The stromal cell system can further be divided into cell populations including fibroblasts and mesenchymal stem cells (MSCs). [43] MSCs reside within the marrow cavity, maintain a level of self-renewal, and give rise to cells that can differentiate into various tissue lineages. [44-49] These populations are functionally and phenotypically defined as osteogenic, adipogenic, and chondrogenic cells as well as a host of other cells including those of cardiac and neural lineage. [50-51]

The developmental defects associated with spina bifida should have no negative effects on bone marrow derived MSC functionality and transdifferentiation properties. This phenomenon has been reported by Kicic et al who describe the terminal differentiation of MSCs obtained from a retinal degenerative mouse model from normal and diseased states. [52]

Both populations of cells responded to external stimuli with expected progression of primitive progenitor cell to differentiated progeny. Isaikina et al have reported similar findings in which bone marrow derived MSCs from children with oncohematological diseases expand and function normally. [53] MSCs obtained from different bodily systems function similarly. [52-56] Therefore, this autologous source of cells would be ideal for coerced differentiation into a smooth muscle cell phenotype for subsequent bladder regeneration.

Chapter VII

MSC Multipotentiality and Growth Characteristics

The differentiation potential of the mesenchymal cell system has been widely studied with respect to the mesenchymal connective tissues, in human and other species. [44, 37, 38] Human mesenchymal cells that had been depleted of circulating hematopoietic cells by negative immunoselection with antibodies against monocytes/macrophages (anti-CD14), endothelial cells (anti-CD31), and lymphocytes (anti-CD11a/LFA-1) are shown to coexpress genes characteristic of the osteoblastic lineage (alkaline phosphatase, osteocalcin, and osteopontin) and adipocytic lineage (lipoprotein lipase), indicating that mesenchymal cells were uncommitted precursor cells. [57] Originally, Pittenger et al have reported that adherent bone marrow-derived stromal colonies are pluripotent and capable of differentiation into the osteogenic, chondrogenic, and adipogenic lineages as demonstrated by lineage specific in vitro assays. [44] The stem–like qualities of MSCs coupled with their transdifferentiation properties have also been demonstrated in other cell and tissue systems. Specifically, through the addition of neurotrophic cytokines including human epidermal growth factor (EGF) and basic fibroblast growth factor (bFGF) under quantified media conditions, Long et al demonstrate that MSCs have the ability to differentiate into cells of neural lineage based upon cell phenotyping, morphological appearance, and growth characteristics. [50]

MSCs form characteristic adherent, fibroblast-like colonies when grown in vitro in fetal calf serum and may be expanded to high numbers ex vivo in the presence of various growth factors. [58,59] There is increasing evidence that single-cell derived colonies are morphologically heterogeneous; they contain a mixture of small, rapidly renewing cells as well as larger cells with slower kinetics of self-renewal. [60,61] The proliferative activity of MSC appears to be directly proportional to their potential to differentiate but both cell types are similarly efficient in supporting cultures of HSCs. [61] Detailed studies have shown that in vitro growth of MSC, as with other progenitor cells, proceeds as a three-phase process with an initial lag phase (3–4 days) followed by a rapid expansion and then a subsequent stationary phase. [62-65] The stationary phase is not dependent on cell contact inhibition and re-plating of MSC from the stationary phase allow them to re-enter the same phases for approximately five passages. It has been proposed that the regulation of the different phases could be under the cyclic expression of various gene products.

Chapter VIII

The Potential of MSCs in Regenerative Medicine

The broad category of stem cells has been heavily explored for its potential use in all disciplines of regenerative medicine. In particular, the potential for MSCs to differentiate into bone, fat, cartilage, muscle, and other lineages has been widely shown. [44, 51, 66] It has been hypothesized that MSCs may target sites of injury, where they then differentiate based on available signals in the surrounding tissue. While these cells have the potential to be beneficial to the injured tissue, this recruitment may also be pathological in nature, as suspected for atherosclerotic plaques. [67, 68] Given the potential beneficial nature of MSCs and the possible utility of these cells for diagnostic applications, there has been a recent interest in investigating the means and stimuli by which recruitment of pre-differentiated MSCs to a tissue site occurs. The advent of transgenic mice and rats constitutively expressing visible reporter genes has allowed for easy tracking of transplanted stem cells in neural and other systems. [69] MSCs in particular have found wide application towards interrogating repair/integration processes in a variety of systems, notably pancreatic, ocular, olfactory, renal, and vascular. [70-81] Notably, MSCs are not universally recruited to all of these tissue systems under every tested condition. Rather, the most noticeable trend is that MSCs are most frequently found to be recruited to injury sites, consistent with their potential to differentiate into inflammatory cells and other lineages. [82] In previous studies investigating the mechanisms of muscle regeneration, the interrelationship between multipotent MSCs and existing muscle cells has been examined in some detail. MSCs have been shown to progress to satellite cells in skeletal muscle and then to mature muscle fibers but do not replenish muscle "side populations," BMSC adoption of muscle phenotype has also been observed through fusion to existing muscle cells. [83-88] As also noted in other tissue systems, labeled MSCs are quickly observed at skeletal muscle injury sites throughout the early stages of recovery, but are only retained in small numbers over long periods, after conversion to satellite cells. [86] Other studies specific to the role of MSCs in SMC regeneration have focused almost exclusively on vascular smooth muscle tissue rather than visceral smooth muscle as found in the bladder. These have demonstrated MSC presence near sites of angiogenesis following arterial ligation, but with no direct incorporation into the neovessels. [81] MSCs have also been extensively found at sites of intimal hyperplasia, both in a cuff-injury model [67] and in vein grafts. [81] These studies on vascular smooth muscle regeneration form the closest link to gaining information regarding BMSC participation in other smooth muscle regeneration.

Chapter IX

Bone Marrow Cells and Bladder Regeneration

There have been several reports using labeled whole bone marrow cells to study their role in bladder regeneration. A variety of biomaterials commonly used for bladder repair were evaluated to determine the functionality of whole bone marrow cells in a bladder regenerative setting. [89] These materials were inserted subcutaneously in the backs of chimeric C57BL/6 mice that had received bone marrow transplants from donors expressing β-galactosidase (scaffolds were not placed anywhere in the urinary tract in this study). The authors found that beyond the initial infiltration of β-gal$^+$ cells (due to inflammatory response), a substantially greater number of MSCs was found in SIS, urinary bladder submucosa (UBS), and PLGA$^+$UBS than in PLGA, collagen I, or the sham control. The authors concluded that scaffold content did influence MSC infiltration and differentiation, but acknowledged that the mechanisms driving this action remained unclear. Based on the limited work above, we now know that a thorough understanding of MSC involvement in bladder reconstruction is vital for several reasons: (1) to document and understand the role of MSCs present in the regenerative process, (2) to potentially exploit MSC multipotency at the site of regeneration, and (3) to understand and reduce any pathogenic muscle formation.

Within the bone marrow cavity, phenotypically specific populations of marrow stem cells have been found to be uncommitted precursor cells capable of multi-cell differentiation. The plastic nature of these bone marrow cells can be exploited within the context of bladder regeneration. Experimental data demonstrated by Kanematsu et al further exemplifies the use of bone marrow cells when utilizing a bladder augmentation model. [90]

The bone marrow transplantation of chimeric eGFP$^+$ rats into wild type recipients that were augmented with bladder acellular matrix (BAM) resulted in positive eGFP expression at two weeks post transplant with a minor population that were both eGFP$^+$/SMA$^+$. However, at 12 weeks post transplant, a larger proportion of cells become eGFP$^+$/SMA$^+$ within the graft. This suggests that a component of the marrow cells was able to home to the site of injury and initiate the regenerative process. An additional study that exemplifies the use of specific populations of MSCs defined by cell surface antigens is the work by Sharma et al. [26] Data from this study indicate that bladder reconstitution occurs more rapidly using epitope defined bone marrow derived MSCs that have been seeded upon a novel elastomeric compound compared to sham or unseeded control animals in a nude rat bladder augmentation model. These cell seeded scaffolds maintained high levels of protein expression of bladder smooth muscle markers and also the formation of smooth muscle bundles by typical found in mature bladder as determined by Trichrome staining. This study further demonstrates the utility of specific bone marrow cells for bladder regeneration. [26] The Sharma and Kanematsu studies both indicate that there exist cellular constituents of the bone marrow that play a crucial role in the regenerative process of the bladder, although those components are not completely understood. The use of an extremely well defined population of mesenchymal stem cells that are proven to be highly plastic in nature and have the ability of differentiating into known lineages such as adipose, osteogenic, and chondrogenic cells appear to be better suited than whole bone marrow cells due to the potential of introducing immune cells into a bladder regenerative setting. However, these studies need to be continued in order to demonstrate increased physiological function of regenerated bladders upon completion of the regenerative process.

Chapter X

Endothelial Progenitor Cells for Vascular Growth

Sources of proangiogenic endothelial progenitor cells (EPCs) arise from the adult bone marrow and are believed to support the integrity of the vascular endothelium. [91-93] Derived from primitive hemangioblasts, EPCs develop within the blood islands of the yolk sac during embryogenesis followed by further development in the fetal liver and subsequently the adult bone marrow. Upon mobilization from the bone marrow, EPCs home to sites of vascular injury and contribute to wound healing or organ regeneration via angiogenesis or neovascularization. Blood vessel development is a regulated process involving the proliferation, migration, and remodeling of endothelial cells (ECs) from adjacent pre-existing blood vessels or following differentiation of EPCs or angioblasts from mesodermal precursors (vasculogenesis). EPCs were originally thought to be present only during embryonic development. However, accumulating evidence in the past several years suggests that they can persist into adult life. This has generated interest in the use of EPCs for neovascularization for regenerative medicine. Although the precise differentiation pathway of an immature EPC to a mature EC is undefined, $CD34^+/CD133^+$ bone marrow derived EPCs have been shown to represent a population of cells that are capable of initiating a neovascularizing or an angiogenic response upon vascular insult (CD133 is a subset population of CD34). [94, 95] The use of EPCs in tissue engineering has been demonstrated by multiple laboratories. Fang et al [96] describe a series of experiments in which decellularized porcine aortic heart valves were seeded with EPCs that were obtained from cord blood. The resulting data obtained demonstrated that EPCs can endothelialize the decellularized matrix to create functional tissue-engineered heart valves, which may then be preconditioned in a bioreactor prior to clinical implantation. Ghajar et al [97] further demonstrate the use of endothelial progenitor cells in a regenerative medicine setting. In this study, endothelial cells are tested for their ability to undergo angiogenesis once seeded upon fibrin matrices. Although the angiogeneic program is initiated in this setting with cytokine treatment, the addition of MSCs upon the matrices increase vascular network formation 7-fold. The resultant data suggest the synergistic effect of MSCs with endothelial cells enhances the neo-angiogenic process. Since the representative fraction of EPCs in the bone marrow is small, ex vivo expansion of these cells with growth factors such as VEGF, bFGF, and IGF-1 would provide large quantities of cells that could then be purified according to their cell surface markers [94, 96, 98] Pro-angiogenic growth factors VEGF, bFGF, and IGF-1 are required for the expansion and development of primitive vasculature in our bladder regeneration model. Therefore, the neo-angiogenic potential of EPCs could be exploited by culturing these cells either upon scaffolds or upon matrices that have been coated with nano-particles or signaling epitopes capable of delivering growth factors. This would potentially create an environment that is conducive for vasculature growth which in turn will allow for the nourishment of the newly formed smooth muscle layer within the bladder wall of a neurogenic bladder.

Chapter XI

Neural Progenitor/Stem Cells

With the identification of neural stem and progenitor cells (NSCs and NPCs, respectively), the possibilities of deriving functional neural tissue from these cells become one step closer to clinical applicability. NSCs were initially isolated and characterized in the early 1990s by Reynolds and Weiss. [99] Putative NSCs were isolated from the adult mouse brain striatum and stimulated with epidermal growth factor in order to promote terminal differentiation of cells into neurons and glial cells, specifically astrocytes. Cells under stimulation expressed the neuroepithelial marker nestin and displayed antibody reactivity to two key neurotransmitters, namely gamma amino butyric acid (GABA) and substance P within an in vivo setting. Further analyses also yielded morphological structures highly analogous to normal, functioning neurons. This pivotal study argued against the traditional dogma that neurogenesis ceases after birth and that damaged brain tissue could not be repaired by internal mechanisms. This lead the way to several other studies that revealed that the identification and isolation of NPCs, which are a subtype of NSCs, from both the central nervous system (CNS) [100,102] and peripheral nervous system (PNS) [103] as well as non-neurogenic regions such as the spinal cord [104] is the focus of research effort to combat neural disorders. [100-104] Data generated from a wide breadth of disciplines has demonstrated the utility of these cells within in vivo models. Prajerova et al describe the terminal differentiation of NPCs into neurons after transplantation into the cortical region of a rat that had undergone photochemical lesion induction resulting in a cerebral infarction. [105] Immunohistochemical analyses for terminally differentiated neuronal markers of transplanted NPCs (one week post transplant) revealed the expression of DCX, β-tubulin III, MAP-2, NeuN and neurofilaments. Further electrophysiological testing of acute brain slices using the patch-clamp technique in whole-cell configurations revealed statistically significant action potentials generated by NPCs as compared to the control sample which consisted of an intact rat cortex sample. These findings suggest that NPCs can be induced to differentiate towards mature neural cells within the appropriate environment. Although brain and spinal tissue are ideal sources for NSCs/NPCs, these sources are fairly inaccessible in clinical setting since they would result in severe consequences of the host in which there were procured. Alternative sources of NSCs/NPCs include those obtained from fetal tissue. Human fetal CNS derived NSCs have demonstrated remarkable potency in several in vivo settings. Studies by Kelly et al reveal the injection of neurospheres derived from NSCs can survive, migrate and differentiate into cells of neural origin and repopulate CNS tissue within the context of an ischemic rat cerebral cortex model. [106] The applications of this study were taken several steps further and applied to a disease model of infantile neuronal ceroid lipofuscinosis (INCL). [107] INCL is a neurodegenerative disease caused by a mutation in the CLN1 gene resulting in aberrant expression of the lysosomal enzyme palmitoyl protein thioesterase-1 (PPT1) which is fatal. [107-109] The PPT1 deficiency causes CNS neural degeneration accompanied by the accumulation of lipofuscin byproducts. PPT1 knockout mice grafted with human NSCs showed marked improvement in PPT1 expression levels with neuroprotection of affected hippocampal and cortical neurons and decreased levels of lipofuscin leading to a delay in motor coordination loss. The results of these studies paved the way for a phase I clinical trial for the juvenile form of neuronal ceroid lipofuscinosis (JNCL or Batten disease) to assess the safety of utilizing fetal human NSCs in this specific clinical setting. Data derived from this trial demonstrated that patients were able to tolerate multiple doses of NSCs which engrafted and survived in various regions of the brain more than one year post transplantation under immunosuppressive therapies. [110, 111]

Although bona fide NSCs have not been utilized in a bladder regenerative setting to date, one report utilizing neuronal-glial restricted precursors facilitated the mild improvement in bladder physiological function.[112] Temeltas et al incorporated the neural-glial cells in a spinal cord injury model of a rat where baseline urodynamic parameters including bladder pressure, capacity, mean contraction amplitude, and mean voiding pressure were all slightly better than control animals.[112] Though this is only one report describing the utility of NSCs derivatives, the field of bladder neuroregeneration is in its embryonic stages and needs to further be explored perhaps in the conjunction with nanomaterials and "smart" scaffolds.

Chapter XII

Embryonic Stem Cells

The derivation of pluripotent stem cells from the developing embryo has created an avenue for pediatric bladder tissue engineering that was not previously available. The identification and characterization of embryonic stem (ES) cells from mouse embryoblasts in the early 1980s paved the way towards the isolation of human ES cells [113,114] although it was known in the early 1960s that cells taken from teratocarcinoma cells could give rise to embryonal carcinoma stem cells capable of trans-germ layer terminal differentiation. [115] ES cells are derived from the inner cell mass of the developing blastocyst several days post-fertilization and are capable of unlimited, undifferentiated proliferation in vitro. [113,114] The ES cells are characteristically stromal in appearance and grow into clusters once placed upon mouse feeder layers typically consisting of embryonic fibroblasts. These feeder layers provide the nutrients and growth factors required for growth and expansion of ES cells. [113, 114] These seminal mouse studies demonstrate that single cell entities sub-cloned from ES cell cultures gave rise to differentiated cell types of all three germ layers. Almost two decades following this landmark discovery, Thompson et al describe the isolation of the first human ES cells. [116] Human ES cells were similarly derived from the blastocyst stage of a human embryo and produced pluripotent cell lines capable of differentiating into derivates of all three germ layers including cartilage, bone, smooth muscle, and striated muscle (mesoderm); intestinal epithelium (endoderm); neural epithelium, embryonic ganglia, and stratified squamous epithelium (ectoderm). The human ES cells also expressed high levels of markers consistent of embryonic lineages but not more differentiated cell types while concurrently expressing high levels of the enzyme telomerase, a strong indicator of cellular aging. [116-118] Since the publication of these important findings, there have been hundreds of research articles dedicated to the elucidation of mechanisms involved with human ES cell differentiation; the potential utilization of human ES cells in a regenerative medicine setting, as well as studies addressing the disease aspects of human ES cells.[119-124] More recently, the first human clinical trials utilizing human ES cells to treat acute spinal cord injury has now gone into effect. Along with the unlimited potential that these cells possess, there are also ethical concerns in which the manner these cells are obtained. Pro-life proponents have argued that the destruction of a human embryo for scientific endeavors is synonymous with murder and ES cell harvesting is prohibited by laws in many countries [125-127]. Meanwhile, scientists argue the antithesis and support the notion that these cells have the potential to positively affect many lives afflicted by disease hence research utilizing ES cells should be explored. The moral and ethical conundrums associated with this topic will continue to rage. A recently described alternative method of obtaining embryonic stem cells without embryonic destruction was put forth by Klimanskaya http://www.nature.com/nprot/journal/v2/n8/abs/nprot. 2007. 274.html-a1 et al. [128] Single blastomeres that were removed from embryos via techniques utilized in pre-implantation genetic diagnoses were cultured in vitro in order to recreate the inner cell mass environment. Cell lines derived from this process demonstrated a normal karyotype with the expression of pluripotent protein markers. These cells were also capable of differentiating into all three germ layers. Further studies by Chung et al corroborated these findings. [129] Lastly, of great concern is the potential of the ES cells to generate a substantial immunological response by a immunocompetent host when utilized in a clinical setting. Studies by Swijnenburg et al describe the destruction of transplanted human ES cells by a massive influx of $CD4^+$ T cells as well as infiltration of inflammatory cells leading to the subsequent rejection of the transplanted human ES cells. [130] Immunosuppressive therapies employed within this study to combat the immune response suggest that human ES cells can survive longer when these therapies are present. Extrapolating this data to a clinical environment would suggest that a patient receiving therapeutic ES cells would most likely require immunosuppressive maintenance for an extended period of time opening up the possibility to secondary infections. Hence, autologous cell sources would be ideal for bladder engineering purposes to avoid such situations.

Recently, several research groups have utilized ES cells in an attempt to recreate functional bladder tissue. Oottamasathien et al and Thomas et al describe the creation of an in vivo tissue recombination model in which fetal bladder mesenchyme was utilized as an induction agent to drive mouse ES cells into bladder tissue components including urothelium and smooth muscle cells as demonstrated by antibody staining of uroplakins and smooth muscle α actin, respectively, while simultaneously eliminating the formation of teratomas. [131,132] These studies also yielded information with regards to protein expression patterns dictated by temporal-spatial relationships identifying potential markers of bladder tissue development. A second group studied the formation of bladder tissue from a population of cells taken from post fertilized primordial germ cells, a derivative of embryoid body cells initially taken from the inner cell mass. [133-135] Data from these studies exemplify the pluripotent characteristics of these cells and their abilities to terminally differentiate into bladder tissue wall components with complete bladder regeneration 28 days post implantation within the context of a nude rat bladder augmentation model. Although the aforementioned studies provide a pivotal foundation for the use of ES cells in bladder regenerative medicine, additional data providing evidence that ES cells can be used to create a three-dimensional organ using smart scaffolding materials would lead the field one step further in creating a physiological functional bladder for replacement therapies.

Chapter XIII

Induced Pluripotent Stem Cells

The ethical controversy associated with ES cells provided fuel for researchers to explore other cellular avenues in order to attempt to identify sources of pluripotent stem cells. The knowledge that somatic cell nuclear transfer into oocytes produced embryonic-like cell states begged the question as to what specific factors could play a role in the cellular transformation. Through a highly selective elimination process, four factors were found to be crucial in the reprogramming of cells into a pluripotent state analogous to ES cells. In 2006, the group led by Shinya Tanaka and colleagues produced the first generation of induced pluripotent stem cells (iPS) from mouse embryonic and adult fibroblasts with the addition of the now famous cocktail of transcription factors including Oct3/4, Sox2, c-Myc, and Klf4. [136] These cells retained embryonic like characteristics in which they were able to form cells of all three germ layers, proliferate indefinitely without losing their pluripotency, were also able to form teratomas upon injection into animal models and other salient features which are all hallmark traits of ES cells. This study set the groundwork for the creation of iPS cells of human derivation as described by Takahashi et al and Yu et al. [137, 138] Following similar protocols, each group demonstrated the insertion of different sets of inducing factors into human adult somatic cells. While the Yamanaka group utilized the same set of factors previously described in the murine system, Yu et al chose OCT4, SOX2, NANOG, and LIN28 based upon their initial strategies to identify pluripotent factors suggesting that there may be different combinations or yet to be identified factors (possibly tissue specific) that may play roles the creation of the pluripotent state. Initial studies have since led to a myriad of other studies focusing on specific cell type and disease states.[139-146] Although the use of iPS cells is used in a variety of regenerative medicine based schemes, those pertaining to the regeneration of bladder tissue are currently lacking with no relevant data to date. As the field of iPS cells expands, there are many possible routes in which these cells can be assessed in a bladder regenerative setting as to create the four basic components of the bladder that include the luminal urothelial lining of the bladder, the smooth muscle component, the vasculature and the neural networks required for proper physiological function. The cell sources that have been previously described are but a few potential candidates for urological regenerative medicine.

Chapter XIV

Scaffold Material Selection

Previous work by bioengineers has demonstrated that the choice of scaffold material strongly influences tissue regeneration. Biologically-derived materials offer many similarities to native ECM. These substrates are typically highly porous, and are composed of a variety of structural proteins, glycosaminoglycans, and proteoglycans, as well as other bioactive components such as growth factors. SIS is a porcine-derived matrix, chemically and mechanically processed from intestinal tissue to remove cellular components while retaining a highly collagenous matrix and many growth factors such as bFGF, TGF-β, and VEGF. [147] Other bladder-derived materials, such as BAM grafts [148, 149] have similar properties to SIS and have been shown to also promote variable degrees of bladder regeneration. However, due to the inconsistent nature of SIS and other biological scaffolds, results are variable and not uniform. In comparison to biologically-derived materials, many synthetic polymers are also biocompatible and biodegradable, but are more easily characterized and processed, and more uniform in their content. Poly-α-esters, such as poly(L-lactic acid) (PLLA), poly(glycolic acid) (PGA), and their copolymers (PLGA) are the most commonly used biodegradable synthetic materials. These degrade through hydrolysis to form standard byproducts of cell respiration, and are well known for surgical applications, such as Vicryl sutures. These polymers are easily processed into highly porous fibrous meshes, which support cell in growth and proliferation. Other polymer systems such as polycaprolactones and polyfumarates are also well-documented. [150] For each of these polymers, the scaffold's physical properties can be adjusted through changes in polymer molecular weight or network formation.

Recently, Yang et al have described the synthesis and characterization of a novel family of biodegradable and elastomeric polyesters, the poly(diol citrates). [151, 152] Specifically, [poly(1,8-octanediol-citrate)] otherwise known as POC, has been synthesized by chemically coupling diols of varying length to citric acid in order to form a cross-linked mesh network through unaided polycondensation reactions. Full structural and mechanical evaluation of POC demonstrated that its elastomeric properties can be specifically altered to mimic the pliancy of certain soft tissues [151, 152] such as cartilage and structures with compliance similar to that of small diameter blood vessels. In vitro and in vivo evaluation using cell culture and subcutaneous implantation, respectively, confirmed cell and tissue compatibility. Experimental data which included the seeding of articular chondrocytes from bovine knee upon disk-shaped POC scaffolds demonstrated the ability of the articular chondrocytes to attach to the pore walls within the scaffold, maintain cell phenotype, and form a cartilaginous tissue during the 28 days of culture.[153] Thus, the following unique characteristics of the elastomeric POC would allow for the evaluation of this family of scaffolds as a potential resource for bladder regeneration: 1) a novel synthetic, biodegradable polymer that has been shown to be non-toxic in vivo with negligible release of toxic by-products upon degradation; 2) a relatively short-half life of approximately 5-10 weeks in vivo; 3) a means in which the elasticity modulus of the scaffold can be custom synthesized to mimic elastomeric/mechanical properties of the bladder; and 4) a scaffold that can used as a suture or be sewn in vivo. The control of the elastic component of the scaffold is key to differentiating MSCs into a smooth muscle cell phenotype. Engler et al has demonstrated the effectiveness of utilizing MSCs on surfaces with differing elastic moduli.[154] By changing the elasticity, one can change the differentiation program of MSCs and cause them to form neural, muscle, or bone cells. This is without the prompt of any exogenous growth factor or cytokine treatment. The evaluation of the effects of seeding three dimensional POC scaffolds (with varying elasticity moduli) with MSCs to determine if the POC scaffold can provide a substrate that will drive primitive MSCs into phenotypic SMCs would provide novel insight into the bladder regenerative process.

Biological scaffolds retain extracellular molecules that play pivotal roles in the regenerative process. [30] VEGF and bFGF comprise a small fraction of these molecules that aid in the promotion of vasculature and smooth muscle formation. [34, 35] However, due to the lack of consistency regarding biological characteristics and harvesting techniques, biological scaffolds have failed to produce uniform and consistent results with regard to bladder regeneration. Recent developments in nanotechnology have now allowed for the creation of synthetic scaffolds that have consistent biological properties. Therefore, the utilization of synthetic matrices coated with nanocarriers in the form of peptide amphiphiles (PA) will aid in the recapitulation of the native bladder environment. This is accomplished through the strategic incorporation of PA expressing heparin binding motifs that are capable of recruiting tissue growth promoting factors such as VEGF and bFGF. [155] Synthetic chemistry techniques will allow us to create scaffolds that are highly reproducible, capable of providing biologic signals for tissue growth and development, and reproduce the elastic nature of the bladder to assist in overcoming deficiencies of bladder regeneration.

There still remains a great clinical need to further elucidate strategies for bladder regeneration. Parameters greatly affecting the outcome of bladder regeneration including choice of cell type, tissue vascularization, and scaffold design. The choice of cell source is imperative since this cell population must be able to recapitulate physiological function of native bladder cells and should be autologous in nature to avoid unwanted immune responses. The inadequate vascularization of regenerated tissue often seen in grafted tissue samples needs to be overcome through the use of specific cell types that are able to robustly promote angiogenesis. Lastly, scaffold design and implementation is vital for proper growth and differentiation of seeded target cells. The shortcomings of previous studies can be overcome through the use of non-diseased autologous sources of MSCs and EPCs derived from the bone to promote bladder regeneration and angiogenesis, respectively. Through the synergistic effects of MSCs and EPCs with novel nanodesigned bioscaffolds, functional bladder regeneration is a realistic goal.

Chapter XV

Controlled Delivery of Growth Factors from Scaffolds Enhances Tissue Regeneration

Successful repopulation of tissue engineering scaffolds requires good initial cell attachment, subsequent proliferation throughout the scaffold, and eventual control over induction of cell differentiation and phenotype expression. Growth factors such as VEGF, PDGF, bFGF, TGF-β, BMP, and others are among the signaling proteins that appear to have the greatest control over tissue reintegration with scaffolds and restoration of specialized function. Two of these growth factors, VEGF and bFGF, have significance in bladder regeneration, where muscle growth and neovascularization have been found to be deficient. bFGF has been shown to promote smooth muscle growth and differentiation, while both bFGF and VEGF induce angiogenesis in developing tissues. [156] The general concept of supplementing synthetic scaffolds with growth factors has been applied to many tissue systems, including hepatic, orthopedic, nervous, vascular, and urologic systems, among others. [156-161] However, the protected and controlled delivery of growth factors to the bladder has not been widely explored. We will utilize recent advances in nanotechnology to control local growth factor delivery to better understand temporal effects on cell differentiation as well as attempt to make synthetic scaffolds more biologic in nature.

Chapter XVI

The Use of Nanotechnology with Self-Assembling Matrices Provides an Alternative Method of Growth Factor Delivery

Self-assembling molecules have been investigated for use as biomaterials. [162] These systems rely on electrostatic interactions, hydrogen bonding, and amphiphilicity to create vesicles, micelles, tubes, and more complicated structures. Examples of supramolecular organization are seen throughout nature, such as in the noncovalent assembly of phospholipids into bilayers and vesicles. On a larger scale, the organization of collagen into fibers and bundles employs similar non-covalent interactions between assemblies. Unlike many conventional polymeric biomaterials, self-assembling molecules can be injected into a site in solution, and then triggered to assemble via pH change, ionic changes, or aggregation with biomacromolecules. In some cases, cells can be embedded within the self-assembling molecules as they gel, providing a useful way to immobilize cells within a site of interest. [163-165] Such molecules could also be gelled within the pores of a traditional polymeric scaffold, providing additional structural support for subsequent transplantation into the host.

Chapter XVII

Self-Assembling Nanomolecules

In their most general form, peptide amphiphiles (PAs) have a hydrophobic alkyl tail and a hydrophilic peptide segment. These molecules can be triggered to self-assemble in aqueous solution, via pH or ionic gradient, burying the hydrophobic tails within the center of nanofiber aggregates. The fiber diameters range from 6-8 nm, with lengths of 500 nm or greater. The nanofibers display a desired peptide epitope on their peripheries, for recognition by cell receptors, or for binding to other biomolecules. The nanofibers entangle to form self-supporting gels in aqueous solution, at concentrations as low as 0.5 wt. %. PA solutions often gel quickly in vivo after exposure to gel the soluble macromolecules present in many extracellular fluids. This gelation has been demonstrated with spinal cord fluid, ocular fluids, and synovial fluids by the Stupp Research Group who are pioneers in the field on nano-based self assembling molecules.[165]

Chapter XVII

Self-Assembling Nanomolecules

In their most general form, peptide amphiphiles (PAs) have a hydrophobic alkyl tail and a hydrophilic peptide segment. These molecules can be triggered to self-assemble in aqueous solution, via pH or ionic gradient, burying the hydrophobic tails within the center of nanofiber aggregates. The fiber diameters range from 6-8 nm, with lengths of 500 nm or greater. The nanofibers display a desired peptide epitope on their peripheries, for recognition by cell receptors, or for binding to other biomolecules. The nanofibers entangle to form self-supporting gels in aqueous solution, at concentrations as low as 0.5 wt. %. PA solutions often gel quickly in vivo after exposure to gel the soluble macromolecules present in many extracellular fluids. This gelation has been demonstrated with spinal cord fluid, ocular fluids, and synovial fluids by the Stupp Research Group who are pioneers in the field on nano-based self assembling molecules.[165]

Chapter XVIII

PA Molecules for Growth Factor Delivery

In vivo, growth factors are known to bind reversibly to structural proteins within the ECM. These growth factors are released via direct interaction from cells, or via passive diffusion, enabling eventual paracrine or autocrine signaling. While other tissue engineering matrices require covalent tethering of growth factors, PA molecules can be flexibly designed to bind growth factors via non-covalent interactions.

Heparin is a highly-sulfated polysaccharide, known partially for its ability to bind and activate growth factors such as VEGF and bFGF through interaction with their heparin-binding domains. Loss of the heparin-binding carboxyl-terminal domain of VEGF has been shown to significantly reduce its proliferative effects on endothelium. [166] A pattern of sequence organization for heparin binding has been identified by other researchers, by examining the binding sites of a variety of heparin-binding proteins. [167] Their consensus sequences of –XBBXBX– and –XBBBXXBX–, where X is representative of a hydrophobic amino acid, and B is a basic amino acid, have already been implemented as the terminal epitope of a PA system. By this method, heparin molecules bind non-covalently to PA molecules, and growth factors bind non-covalently to the attached heparin.

Chapter XIX

Differentiation of Neural Progenitor Cells with IKVAV Presenting Nanofibers

Signaling molecules play a crucial role in the maturation of progenitor cells but this need not occur in an in vivo environment. Silva et al eloquently demonstrate the use of peptide amphiphile (PA) technology that incorporates the laminin pentapeptide epitope isoleucine-lysine-valine-alanine-valine (IKVAV) that is known to promote neurite sprouting and to direct neurite growth. [165, 168-172] NPCs encapsulated into IKVAV-PA containing gels were grown on glass slides and expressed proteins of mature neuronal lineage at day 7. When compared to a laminin coated control slides, the IKVAV-PA system contained a 20 fold greater number of neuronal cells with very few contaminating astrocytes. This data suggests that the presence of the IKVAV sequence allows for greater specificity for neuronal cell differentiation. Furthermore, Nakamura et al provide valuable insight into the angiogenic promoting role of the IKVAV sequence. [173] A chick chorioallantoic membrane model seeded with an artificial extracellular matrix displaying the IKVAV sequence promoted vascular formation to greater levels than a collagen binding domain only control sample which were statistically significant. These data taken together, along with data generated from the Rivera study [174] which describe the neural promoting activities of MSCs, indicate that the coupling of the IKVAV sequence to novel elastomers such as POC may also provide an alternate means to create an environment conducive for efficient regeneration of functional bladder tissue.

Chapter XX

Summary

Data from multiple laboratories spanning greater than a decade of research have not been able to conclusively demonstrate a bladder with sustained normal physiological function following regenerative therapies. Current therapies still suffer from either the long term ramifications of surgical intervention or poor outcomes when tissue engineering techniques have been applied. Therefore, there still remains a great clinical need to further elucidate strategies utilizing easily obtainable cell sources in combination with synthetic scaffolds that can be synthesized to function to mimic biological scaffold. The shortcomings regarding bladder regeneration involve the choice of cell type, tissue vascularization, scaffold design and the incorporation of functional neural circuits. The multipotentiality of bone marrow derived MSCs, ESCs, iPS cells described in clearly demonstrates that these primitive cells can be coaxed into a variety of functional cell lineages that could possibly be used to create functional bladder tissue. Key attributes of MSCs, ESCs, and iPS cells are their ability to expand to high numbers ex vivo while still retaining their multipotency which will be necessary in a bladder regenerative setting. Vascularization of the developing tissue can also be provided from autologous bone marrow derived EPCs. These cells have been shown to promote the formation of fully functional vasculature capable of nourishing developing tissue. Nanodesigned scaffolds and novel elastomeric compounds will act as a delivery vehicles to supply structural support as well as growth factors/signaling epitopes needed for bladder development. Through the combination of nanotechnology/materials science and novel attributes of stem cell biology, it may be possible to attain the elusive goal of a fully functional bladder that could be used for patients suffering from developmental or acquired defects including trauma, bladder cancer, and spina bifida.

[49] Wang D, Park JS, Chu JS, Krakowski A, Luo Proteomic profiling of bone marrow mesenchymal stem cells upon transforming growth factor beta1 stimulation. *J Biol Chem.* 2004, 279(42):43725-43734.
[50] Long X, Olszewski M, Huang W, Kletzel M. Neural cell differentiation in vitro from adult human bone marrow mesenchymal stem cells. *Stem Cells Dev.* 2005, 14(1):65-69.
[51] Toma C, Pittenger MF, Cahill KS, Byrne BJ, Kessler PD. Human mesenchymal stem cells differentiate to a cardiomyocyte phenotype in the adult murine heart. *Circulation.* 2002, 105(1):93-98.
[52] Kicic A, Hall CM, Shen WY, Rakoczy PE. Are stem cell characteristics altered by disease state? *Stem Cells Dev.* 2005, 14(1):15-28.
[53] Isaikina Y, Kustanovich A, Svirnovski A. Growth kinetics and self-renewal of human mesenchymal stem cells derived from bone marrow of children with oncohematological diseases during expansion in vitro. *Exp Oncol.* 2006, 28(2):146-151.
[54] Caplan A, Dennis J. Genetically Linked Scientists: The One-Two Punch For NFATp Knockout. *Journal of Experimental Medicine* 2000, 191(1) 1-4.
[55] Tatebe M, Nakamura R, Kagami H, Okada K, Ueda M. Differentiation of transplanted mesenchymal stem cells in a large osteochondral defect in rabbit. *Cytotherapy.* 2005, 7(6):520-530.
[56] Adachi N, Ochi M, Deie M, Ito Y. Transplant of mesenchymal stem cells and hydroxyapatite ceramics to treat severe osteochondral damage after septic arthritis of the knee. *J Rheumatol.* 2005, 32(8):1615-1618.
[57] Le Blanc K, Pittenger M. Mesenchymal stem cells: progress toward promise. *Cytotherapy.* 2005, 7(1):36-45.
[58] Shahdadfar A, Frønsdal K, Haug T, Reinholt F, Brinchmann J. *In Vitro Expansion of Human Mesenchymal Stem Cells: Choice of Serum Is a Determinant of Cell Proliferation, Differentiation, Gene Expression, and Transcriptome Stability Stem Cells* 2005, 23(9): 1357-1366.
[59] Beyer Nardi N, da Silva Meirelles L. Mesenchymal stem cells: isolation, in vitro expansion and characterization. *Handb Exp Pharmacol.* 2006, (174):249-282.
[60] Gottschling S, Saffrich R, Seckinger A, Krause U, Horsch K, Miesala K, Ho AD. Human mesenchymal stromal cells regulate initial self-renewing divisions of hematopoietic progenitor cells by a beta1-integrin-dependent mechanism. *Stem Cells.* 2007 Mar, 25(3):798-806.

[61] Li N, Feugier P, Serrurrier B, Latger-Cannard V, Lesesve JF, Stoltz JF, Eljaafari A. Human mesenchymal stem cells improve ex vivo expansion of adult human CD34+ peripheral blood progenitor cells and decrease their allostimulatory capacity. *Exp Hematol.* 2007, 35(3):507-515.

[62] Kang TJ, Yeom JE, Lee HJ, Rho SH, Han H, Chae GT. Growth kinetics of human mesenchymal stem cells from bone marrow and umbilical cord blood. *Acta Haematol.* 2004, 112(4):230-233.

[63] Bruder SP, Jaiswal N, Haynesworth SE. Growth kinetics, self-renewal, and the osteogenic potential of purified human mesenchymal stem cells during extensive subcultivation and following cryopreservation. *J Cell Biochem.* 1997, 64(2):278-294.

[64] Gordeladze C, Noel D. Tissue engineering through autologous mesenchymal stem cells. *Curr Opin Biotech* 2004, 15(5): 406-410.

[65] Krampera M, Pasini A, Rigo A, Scupoli MT, Tecchio C, Malpeli G, Scarpa A, Dazzi F, Pizzolo G, Vinante F HB-EGF/HER-1 signaling in bone marrow mesenchymal stem cells: inducing cell expansion and reversibly preventing multilineage differentiation. *Blood.* 2005, 106(1):59-66.

[66] Sato Y, Araki H, Kato J, Nakamura K, Kawano Y, Kobune M, Sato T, Miyanishi K, Takayama T, Takahashi M, Takimoto R, Iyama S, Matsunaga T, Ohtani S, Matsuura A, Hamada H, Niitsu Y. Human mesenchymal stem cells xenografted directly to rat liver are differentiated into human hepatocytes without fusion. *Blood.* 2005,106(2):756-763.

[67] Xu, Y, Arai H, Zhuge X, Sano H, Murayama T, Yoshimoto M. Heike T, Nakahata T, Nishikawa S, Kita T, Yokode M. Role of bone marrow-derived progenitor cells in cuff-induced vascular injury in mice. *Arter Thromb Vas Bio* 2004, 24(3): 477-482.

[68] Saiura A, Sata M, Washida M, Sugawara Y, Hirata Y, Nagai R, Makuuchi M. Little evidence for cell fusion between recipient and donor-derived cells. *J of Surg Res* 2003, 113(2): 222-227.

[69] Mothe AJ, Kulbatski I, van Bendegem RL, Lee L, Kobayashi E, Keating A, Tator CH. Analysis of green fluorescent protein expression in transgenic rats for tracking transplanted neural stem/progenitor cells. *J Histo Cyto* 2005, 53(10):1215-1226.

[70] Lechner A, Yang YG, Blacken RA, Wang L, Nolan AL, Habener JF. No evidence for significant transdifferentiation of bone marrow into pancreatic beta-cells in vivo. *Diabetes* 2004, 53(3):616-623.

[71] Nakamura T, Ishikawa F, Sonoda KH, Hisatomi T, Qiao H, Yamada J, Fukata M, Ishibashi T, Harada M, Kinoshita S. Characterization and distribution of bone marrow-derived cells in mouse cornea. *Investigative Oph Vis Sci* 2005, 46 (2):497-503.

[72] Qiao H, Hisatomi T, Sonoda KH, Kura S, Sassa Y, Kinoshita S, Nakamura T, Sakamoto T, Ishibashi T. The characterisation of hyalocytes: the origin, phenotype, and turnover. *Brit J Oph* 2005, 89(4):513-517.

[73] Espinosa-Heidmann DG, Caicedo A, Hernandez EP, Csaky KG, Cousins SW. Bone marrow-derived progenitor cells contribute to experimental choroidal neovascularization. *Investigative Oph Vis Sci* 2003, 44(11):4914-4919.

[74] Espinosa-Heidmann DG, Reinoso MA, Pina Y, Csaky KG, Caicedo A, Cousins SW. Quantitative enumeration of vascular smooth muscle cells and endothelial cells derived from bone marrow precursors in experimental choroidal neovascularization. *Exp Eye Res* 2005, 80(3):369-378.

[75] Sengupta N, Caballero S, Mames RN, Butler JM, Scott EW, Grant MB. The role of adult bone marrow-derived stem cells in choroidal neovascularization. *Investigative Oph Vis Sci* 2003, 44(11):4908-4913.

[76] Takahashi H, Yanagi Y, Tamaki Y, Muranaka K, Usui T, Sata M. Contribution of bone marrow-derived cells to choroidal neovascularization. *Biochemical & Biophysical Res Com* 2004, 320(2):372-375.

[77] Moore BE, Colvin GA, Dooner MS, Quesenberry PJ. Lineage-negative bone marrow cells travel bidirectionally in the olfactory migratory stream but maintain hematopoietic phenotype. *Journal of Cellular Physiology* 2005, 202(1):147-152.

[78] Duffield JS, Park KM, Hsiao LL, Kelley VR, Scadden DT, Ichimura T, Bonventre JV. Restoration of tubular epithelial cells during repair of the postischemic kidney occurs independently of bone marrow-derived stem cells.*J of Clin Invest* 2005, 115(7):1743-1755.

[79] Lin F, Moran A, Igarashi P. Intrarenal cells, not bone marrow-derived cells, are the major source for regeneration in postischemic kidney. *Journal of Clinical Investigation* 2005, 115(7):1756-1764.

[80] Zhang L, Freedman NJ, Brian L, Peppel K. Graft-extrinsic cells predominate in vein graft arterialization. *Arter, Thromb Vas Bio* 2004, 24(3):470-476.
[81] Ziegelhoeffer T, Fernandez B, Kostin S, Heil M, Voswinckel R, Helisch A, Schaper W. Bone marrow-derived cells do not incorporate into the adult growing vasculature. *Circ Res* 2004, 94(2):230-238.
[82] Abedi M, Greer DA, Colvin GA, Demers DA, Dooner MS, Harpel JA, Pimentel J, Menon MK, Quesenberry PJ. Tissue injury in marrow transdifferentiation. *Blood Cells Mole Dis* 2004, 32(1):42-46.
[83] Natsu K, Ochi M, Mochizuki Y, Hachisuka H, Yanada S, Yasunaga Y. Allogeneic bone marrow-derived mesenchymal stromal cells promote the regeneration of injured skeletal muscle without differentiation into myofibers. *Tiss Eng* 2004, 10(7-8):1093-1112.
[84] Loscalzo, J. Stem cells and regeneration of the cardiovascular system: facts, fictions, and uncertainties. *Blood Cells Mole Dis* 2004, 32(1):97-99.
[85] LaBarge M, Blau M. Biological progression from adult bone marrow to mononucleate muscle stem cell to multinucleate muscle fiber in response to injury. *Cell* 2002, 111(4), 589-601.
[86] Yoshimoto M, Chang H, Shiota M, Kobayashi H, Umeda K, Kawakami A, Heike T, Nakahata T. Two different roles of purified CD45+c-Kit+Sca-1+Lin- cells after transplantation in muscles. *Stem Cells* 2005, 23(5): 610-618.
[87] Rivier F, Alkan O, Flint AF, Muskiewicz K, Allen PD, Leboulch P, Gussoni E. Role of bone marrow cell trafficking in replenishing skeletal muscle SP and MP cell populations. *J Cell Sci* 2004, 117(Pt 10):1979-1988.
[88] Shi D, Reinecke H, Murry CE, Torok-Storb B. Myogenic fusion of human bone marrow stromal cells, but not hematopoietic cells. *Blood* 2004, 104(1):290-294.
[89] Badylak SF, Park K, Peppas N, McCabe G, Yoder M. Marrow-derived cells populate scaffolds composed of xenogeneic extracellular matrix. *Exp Hem* 2001, 29(11):1310-1318.
[90] Kanematsu A, Yamamoto S, Iwai-Kanai E, Kanatani I, Imamura M, Adam RM, Tabata Y, Ogawa O. Induction of smooth muscle cell-like phenotype in marrow-derived cells among regenerating urinary bladder smooth muscle cells. *Am J Pathol.* 2005, 166(2):565-573.

References

[1] www.nlm.nih.gov/medlineplus/bladderdiseases.html
[2] Clayton DB, Brock JW 3rd, Joseph DB. Urologic management of spina bifida. *Dev Disabil Res Rev.* 2010;16(1):88-95.
[3] de Jong TP, Chrzan R, Klijn AJ, Dik P. Treatment of the neurogenic bladder in spina bifida. *Pediatr Nephrol.* 2008 Jun;23(6):889-896.
[4] Atala A, Bauer SB, Soker S, Yoo JJ, Retik AB. Tissue-engineered autologous bladders for patients needing cystoplasty. *Lancet.* 2006 Apr 15;367(9518):1241-1246.
[5] Andersson KE. Pathways for relaxation of detrusor smooth muscle. *Adv Exp Med Biol.* 1999;462:241-252.
[6] Levin TL, Han B, Little BP. Congenital anomalies of the male urethra. *Pediatr Radiol.* 2007 Sep;37(9):851-862.
[7] Fritsch H, Pinggera GM, Lienemann A, Mitterberger M, Bartsch G, Strasser H. What are the supportive structures of the female urethra? *Neurourol Urodyn.* 2006;25(2):128-134.
[8] Rickard A, Dorokhov N, Ryerse J, Klumpp DJ, McHowat J. Characterization of tight junction proteins in cultured human urothelial cells. *In Vitro Cell Dev Biol Anim.* 2008 Jul-Aug;44(7):261-267.
[9] DeLancey J, Gosling JA, Creed KE, Dixon J, Delmas V, Landon D, Norton P. Gross anatomy and cell biology of the lower urinary tract. *In:Incontinence, SecondInternational Consultation on Incontinence,* edited by Abrams P, Cardozo L, Khoury S, and Wein A. Plymouth, MA: Health Publication, 2002, p.17-82.
[10] Dixon J, Golsing A. Ultrastructure of smooth muscle cells in the urinary system. In: *Ultrastructure of Smooth Muscles,* edited by Motta PM. London: Kluwer Academic, 1990, p.153-169.
[11] Benninghoff 1993 Benninghoff, A.: *Makroskopische Anatomie, Embryologie und Histologie des Menschen.* 15. Auflage. München; Wien; Baltimore: Urban und Schwarzenberg, 1993

[12] Andersson KE, Arner A. Urinary bladder contraction and relaxation: physiology and pathophysiology. *Physiol Rev.* 2004 Jul;84(3):935-986.
[13] Akita K, Sakamoto H, Sato T. Origins and courses of the nervous branches to the male urethral sphincter. *Surg Radiol Anat.* 2003 Nov-Dec;25(5-6):387-392.
[14] Podnar S. Neurophysiology of the neurogenic lower urinary tract disorders. *Clin Neurophysiol.* 2007 Jul;118(7):1423-1437.
[15] Fry CH, Ikeda Y, Harvey R, Wu C, Sui GP. Control of bladder function by peripheral nerves: avenues for novel drug targets. *Urology.* 2004 Mar;63(3 Suppl 1):24-31.
[16] Onishi N, Kiwamoto H, Esa A, Sugiyama T, Paku YC, Kaneko S, Kurita T. *Neurogenic bladder dysfunction due to tethered spinal cord syndrome in adults: report of two cases.* Hinyokika Kiyo, 1989, (35):1229-1234.
[17] Ab E, Dik P, Klijn AJ, van Gool JD, de Jong TP. Detrusor overactivity in spina bifida: how long does it need to be treated? *Neurourol Urodyn.* 2004; 23(7):685-688.
[18] Matsumoto S, Hanai T, Kurita T, Akiyama T. *Phenotypic changes in human bladder smooth muscle cell.* Hinyokika Kiyo. 2003, 49(12):715-719.
[19] Rodó JS, Cáceres FA, Lerena JR, Rossy E. Bladder augmentation and artificial sphincter implantation: urodynamic behavior and effects on continence. *J Pediatr Urol.* 2008 Feb;4(1):8-13.
[20] Cameron AP, Clemens JQ, Latini JM, McGuire EJ. Combination drug therapy improves compliance of the neurogenic bladder.*J Urol.* 2009 Sep;182(3):1062-1067.
[21] Zini L, Yiou R, Lecoeur C, Biserte J, Abbou C, Chopin DK. Tissue engineering in urology. *Ann Urol (Paris).* 2004, 38(6):266-274.
[22] Husmann DA, Snodgrass WT, Koyle MA, Furness PD, Kropp BP, Cheng EY, Kaplan WE, Kramer SA. Ureterocystoplasty: indications for a successful augmentation. *J Urol.* 2004, 171(1):376-380.
[23] Metwalli, A. R., Colvert, J. R., 3rd, Kropp, B. P. Tissue engineering in urology: where are we going? *Curr Urol Rep.* 2003, 4(2):156-163.
[24] Zini L, Yiou R, Lecoeur C, Biserte J, Abbou C, Chopin DK. Tissue engineering in urology. *Ann Urol (Paris).* 2004, 38(6):266-274.

[25] Husmann DA, Snodgrass WT, Koyle MA, Furness PD, Kropp BP, Cheng EY, Kaplan WE, Kramer SA. Ureterocystoplasty: indications for a successful augmentation. *J Urol.* 2004, 171(1):376-380.
[26] Sharma AK, Hota PV, Matoka DJ, Fuller NJ, Jandali D, Thaker H, Ameer GA, Cheng EY. Urinary bladder smooth muscle regeneration utilizing bone marrow derived mesenchymal stem cell seeded elastomeric poly(1,8-octanediol-co-citrate) based thin films. *Biomaterials.* 2010 Aug;31(24):6207-6217.
[27] Bankhead, R. W., Kropp, B. P., Cheng, E. Y.: Evaluation and treatment of children with neurogenic bladders. *J Child Neurol.* 2000, 15(3):141-149.
[28] Cetinel, B. Reconstructive surgery in neuropathic bladder. *Adv Exp Med Biol.* 2003, 539(Pt A):509-533.
[29] http://www.spinabifidaassociation.org
[30] Zhang Y, Kropp BP, Lin HK, Cowan R, Cheng EY. Bladder regeneration with cell-seeded small intestinal submucosa. *Tissue Eng.* 2004, 10(1-2):181-187.
[31] Atala, A. Future perspectives in bladder reconstruction. *Adv Exp Med Biol.* 2003; 539(Pt B):921-940.
[32] Atala, A. Bladder regeneration by tissue engineering. *BJU Int.* 2001, 88(7):765-770.
[33] Oberpenning F, Meng J, Yoo JJ, Atala A. De novo reconstitution of a functional mammalian urinary bladder by tissue engineering. *Nat Biotechnol.* 1999 Feb;17(2):149-155.
[34] Lin HK, Cowan R, Moore P, Zhang Y, Yang Q, Peterson JA Jr, Tomasek JJ, Kropp BP, Cheng EY. Neurogenic cells are different in vitro Characterization of neuropathic bladder smooth muscle cells in culture. *J Urol.* 2004 171(3):1348-1352.
[35] Beqaj SH, Donovan JL, Liu DB, Harrington DA, Alpert SA, Cheng EY. Role of basic fibroblast growth factor in the neuropathic bladder phenotype. *J Urol.* 2005 174(4 Pt 2):1699-1703.
[36] Chen LT, Weiss L. The development of vertebral bone marrow of human fetuses. *Blood.* 1975, 46(3):389-408.
[37] Gilmour JR Normal hematopoiesis in intrauterine and neonatal life. *J Pathol* 53:25, 1941

[38] Escobar MR, Friedman H, Reichard SM. *The reticuloendothelial System: A Comphrehensive Treatise.* Vols 1-10. Plenum, New York, 1979-1988.
[39] Weiss L. Bone marrow, spleen, thymus; lymphatic vessels and lymph nodes. In Weiss L (ed): *Cell and Tissue Biology: A Textbook of Histology.* 6th *Ed.* Urban and Scharzenburg, Baltimore, 1988
[40] Tavassoli M. Marrow adipose cells. Histochemical identification of labile and stable components. *Arch Pathol Lab Med.* 1976, 100(1):16-18.
[41] McCuskey RS, Meineke HA. Studies of the hemopoietic microenvironment. Differences in the splenic microvascular system and stroma between SL-SL d and W-W v anemic mice. *Am J Anat.* 1973, 137(2):187-197.
[42] Weiss L, Chen HT. The organization of hematopoietic cords and vascular sinuses in bone marrow. *Blood Cells* 1975 1:617.
[43] Kolf CM, Cho E, Tuan RS. Mesenchymal stromal cells. Biology of adult mesenchymal stem cells: regulation of niche, self-renewal and differentiation. Arthritis Res Ther. 2007, 9(1):204.
[44] Pittenger MF, Mackay AM, Beck SC, Jaiswal RK, Douglas R, Mosca JD, Moorman MA, Simonetti DW, Craig S, Mars Multilineage potential of adult human mesenchymal stem cells. *Science.* 2;284(5411):143-147.
[45] Jaiswal RK, Jaiswal N, Bruder SP Adult human mesenchymal stem cell differentiation to the osteogenic or adipogenic lineage is regulated by mitogen-activated protein kinase. *J Biol Chem.* 2000, 275(13):9645-9652.
[46] Lee K, Majumdar MK, Buyaner D, Hendricks JK, Pittenger MF, Mosca JD. Human mesenchymal stem cells maintain transgene expression during expansion and differentiation. *Mol Ther.* 20003, 3(6):857-866.
[47] Niemeyer P, Kasten P, Simank HG, Fellenberg J, Seckinger A, Kreuz P, Mehlhorn A, Sudkamp N, Krause U. Transplantation of mesenchymal stromal cells on mineralized collagen leads to ectopic matrix synthesis in vivo independently from prior in vitro differentiation. *Cytotherapy.* 2006;8(4):354-366.
[48] Kim DH, Yoo KH, Choi KS, Choi J, Choi SY, Yang SE, Yang YS, Im HJ, Kim KH, Jung HL, Sung KW, Koo HH. Gene expression profile of cytokine and growth factor during differentiation of bone marrow-derived mesenchymal stem cell. *Cytokine.* 2005, 31(2):119-126

[49] Wang D, Park JS, Chu JS, Krakowski A, Luo Proteomic profiling of bone marrow mesenchymal stem cells upon transforming growth factor beta1 stimulation. *J Biol Chem.* 2004, 279(42):43725-43734.
[50] Long X, Olszewski M, Huang W, Kletzel M. Neural cell differentiation in vitro from adult human bone marrow mesenchymal stem cells. *Stem Cells Dev.* 2005, 14(1):65-69.
[51] Toma C, Pittenger MF, Cahill KS, Byrne BJ, Kessler PD. Human mesenchymal stem cells differentiate to a cardiomyocyte phenotype in the adult murine heart. *Circulation.* 2002, 105(1):93-98.
[52] Kicic A, Hall CM, Shen WY, Rakoczy PE. Are stem cell characteristics altered by disease state? *Stem Cells Dev.* 2005, 14(1):15-28.
[53] Isaikina Y, Kustanovich A, Svirnovski A. Growth kinetics and self-renewal of human mesenchymal stem cells derived from bone marrow of children with oncohematological diseases during expansion in vitro. *Exp Oncol.* 2006, 28(2):146-151.
[54] Caplan A, Dennis J. Genetically Linked Scientists: The One-Two Punch For NFATp Knockout. *Journal of Experimental Medicine* 2000, 191(1) 1-4.
[55] Tatebe M, Nakamura R, Kagami H, Okada K, Ueda M. Differentiation of transplanted mesenchymal stem cells in a large osteochondral defect in rabbit. *Cytotherapy.* 2005, 7(6):520-530.
[56] Adachi N, Ochi M, Deie M, Ito Y. Transplant of mesenchymal stem cells and hydroxyapatite ceramics to treat severe osteochondral damage after septic arthritis of the knee. *J Rheumatol.* 2005, 32(8):1615-1618.
[57] Le Blanc K, Pittenger M. Mesenchymal stem cells: progress toward promise. *Cytotherapy.* 2005, 7(1):36-45.
[58] Shahdadfar A, Frønsdal K, Haug T, Reinholt F, Brinchmann J. *In Vitro Expansion of Human Mesenchymal Stem Cells: Choice of Serum Is a Determinant of Cell Proliferation, Differentiation, Gene Expression, and Transcriptome Stability Stem Cells* 2005, 23(9): 1357-1366.
[59] Beyer Nardi N, da Silva Meirelles L. Mesenchymal stem cells: isolation, in vitro expansion and characterization. *Handb Exp Pharmacol.* 2006, (174):249-282.
[60] Gottschling S, Saffrich R, Seckinger A, Krause U, Horsch K, Miesala K, Ho AD. Human mesenchymal stromal cells regulate initial self-renewing divisions of hematopoietic progenitor cells by a beta1-integrin-dependent mechanism. *Stem Cells.* 2007 Mar, 25(3):798-806.

[61] Li N, Feugier P, Serrurrier B, Latger-Cannard V, Lesesve JF, Stoltz JF, Eljaafari A. Human mesenchymal stem cells improve ex vivo expansion of adult human CD34+ peripheral blood progenitor cells and decrease their allostimulatory capacity. *Exp Hematol.* 2007, 35(3):507-515.
[62] Kang TJ, Yeom JE, Lee HJ, Rho SH, Han H, Chae GT. Growth kinetics of human mesenchymal stem cells from bone marrow and umbilical cord blood. *Acta Haematol.* 2004, 112(4):230-233.
[63] Bruder SP, Jaiswal N, Haynesworth SE. Growth kinetics, self-renewal, and the osteogenic potential of purified human mesenchymal stem cells during extensive subcultivation and following cryopreservation. *J Cell Biochem.* 1997, 64(2):278-294.
[64] Gordeladze C, Noel D. Tissue engineering through autologous mesenchymal stem cells. *Curr Opin Biotech* 2004, 15(5): 406-410.
[65] Krampera M, Pasini A, Rigo A, Scupoli MT, Tecchio C, Malpeli G, Scarpa A, Dazzi F, Pizzolo G, Vinante F HB-EGF/HER-1 signaling in bone marrow mesenchymal stem cells: inducing cell expansion and reversibly preventing multilineage differentiation. *Blood.* 2005, 106(1):59-66.
[66] Sato Y, Araki H, Kato J, Nakamura K, Kawano Y, Kobune M, Sato T, Miyanishi K, Takayama T, Takahashi M, Takimoto R, Iyama S, Matsunaga T, Ohtani S, Matsuura A, Hamada H, Niitsu Y. Human mesenchymal stem cells xenografted directly to rat liver are differentiated into human hepatocytes without fusion. *Blood.* 2005,106(2):756-763.
[67] Xu, Y, Arai H, Zhuge X, Sano H, Murayama T, Yoshimoto M. Heike T, Nakahata T, Nishikawa S, Kita T, Yokode M. Role of bone marrow-derived progenitor cells in cuff-induced vascular injury in mice. *Arter Thromb Vas Bio* 2004, 24(3): 477-482.
[68] Saiura A, Sata M, Washida M, Sugawara Y, Hirata Y, Nagai R, Makuuchi M. Little evidence for cell fusion between recipient and donor-derived cells. *J of Surg Res* 2003, 113(2): 222-227.
[69] Mothe AJ, Kulbatski I, van Bendegem RL, Lee L, Kobayashi E, Keating A, Tator CH. Analysis of green fluorescent protein expression in transgenic rats for tracking transplanted neural stem/progenitor cells. *J Histo Cyto* 2005, 53(10):1215-1226.

[70] Lechner A, Yang YG, Blacken RA, Wang L, Nolan AL, Habener JF. No evidence for significant transdifferentiation of bone marrow into pancreatic beta-cells in vivo. *Diabetes* 2004, 53(3):616-623.

[71] Nakamura T, Ishikawa F, Sonoda KH, Hisatomi T, Qiao H, Yamada J, Fukata M, Ishibashi T, Harada M, Kinoshita S. Characterization and distribution of bone marrow-derived cells in mouse cornea. *Investigative Oph Vis Sci* 2005, 46 (2):497-503.

[72] Qiao H, Hisatomi T, Sonoda KH, Kura S, Sassa Y, Kinoshita S, Nakamura T, Sakamoto T, Ishibashi T. The characterisation of hyalocytes: the origin, phenotype, and turnover. *Brit J Oph* 2005, 89(4):513-517.

[73] Espinosa-Heidmann DG, Caicedo A, Hernandez EP, Csaky KG, Cousins SW. Bone marrow-derived progenitor cells contribute to experimental choroidal neovascularization. *Investigative Oph Vis Sci* 2003, 44(11):4914-4919.

[74] Espinosa-Heidmann DG, Reinoso MA, Pina Y, Csaky KG, Caicedo A, Cousins SW. Quantitative enumeration of vascular smooth muscle cells and endothelial cells derived from bone marrow precursors in experimental choroidal neovascularization. *Exp Eye Res* 2005, 80(3):369-378.

[75] Sengupta N, Caballero S, Mames RN, Butler JM, Scott EW, Grant MB. The role of adult bone marrow-derived stem cells in choroidal neovascularization. *Investigative Oph Vis Sci* 2003, 44(11):4908-4913.

[76] Takahashi H, Yanagi Y, Tamaki Y, Muranaka K, Usui T, Sata M. Contribution of bone marrow-derived cells to choroidal neovascularization. *Biochemical & Biophysical Res Com* 2004, 320(2):372-375.

[77] Moore BE, Colvin GA, Dooner MS, Quesenberry PJ. Lineage-negative bone marrow cells travel bidirectionally in the olfactory migratory stream but maintain hematopoietic phenotype. *Journal of Cellular Physiology* 2005, 202(1):147-152.

[78] Duffield JS, Park KM, Hsiao LL, Kelley VR, Scadden DT, Ichimura T, Bonventre JV. Restoration of tubular epithelial cells during repair of the postischemic kidney occurs independently of bone marrow-derived stem cells.*J of Clin Invest* 2005, 115(7):1743-1755.

[79] Lin F, Moran A, Igarashi P. Intrarenal cells, not bone marrow-derived cells, are the major source for regeneration in postischemic kidney. *Journal of Clinical Investigation* 2005, 115(7):1756-1764.

[80] Zhang L, Freedman NJ, Brian L, Peppel K. Graft-extrinsic cells predominate in vein graft arterialization. *Arter, Thromb Vas Bio* 2004, 24(3):470-476.
[81] Ziegelhoeffer T, Fernandez B, Kostin S, Heil M, Voswinckel R, Helisch A, Schaper W. Bone marrow-derived cells do not incorporate into the adult growing vasculature. *Circ Res* 2004, 94(2):230-238.
[82] Abedi M, Greer DA, Colvin GA, Demers DA, Dooner MS, Harpel JA, Pimentel J, Menon MK, Quesenberry PJ. Tissue injury in marrow transdifferentiation. *Blood Cells Mole Dis* 2004, 32(1):42-46.
[83] Natsu K, Ochi M, Mochizuki Y, Hachisuka H, Yanada S, Yasunaga Y. Allogeneic bone marrow-derived mesenchymal stromal cells promote the regeneration of injured skeletal muscle without differentiation into myofibers. *Tiss Eng* 2004, 10(7-8):1093-1112.
[84] Loscalzo, J. Stem cells and regeneration of the cardiovascular system: facts, fictions, and uncertainties. *Blood Cells Mole Dis* 2004, 32(1):97-99.
[85] LaBarge M, Blau M. Biological progression from adult bone marrow to mononucleate muscle stem cell to multinucleate muscle fiber in response to injury. *Cell* 2002, 111(4), 589-601.
[86] Yoshimoto M, Chang H, Shiota M, Kobayashi H, Umeda K, Kawakami A, Heike T, Nakahata T. Two different roles of purified CD45+c-Kit+Sca-1+Lin- cells after transplantation in muscles. *Stem Cells* 2005, 23(5): 610-618.
[87] Rivier F, Alkan O, Flint AF, Muskiewicz K, Allen PD, Leboulch P, Gussoni E. Role of bone marrow cell trafficking in replenishing skeletal muscle SP and MP cell populations. *J Cell Sci* 2004, 117(Pt 10):1979-1988.
[88] Shi D, Reinecke H, Murry CE, Torok-Storb B. Myogenic fusion of human bone marrow stromal cells, but not hematopoietic cells. *Blood* 2004, 104(1):290-294.
[89] Badylak SF, Park K, Peppas N, McCabe G, Yoder M. Marrow-derived cells populate scaffolds composed of xenogeneic extracellular matrix. *Exp Hem* 2001, 29(11):1310-1318.
[90] Kanematsu A, Yamamoto S, Iwai-Kanai E, Kanatani I, Imamura M, Adam RM, Tabata Y, Ogawa O. Induction of smooth muscle cell-like phenotype in marrow-derived cells among regenerating urinary bladder smooth muscle cells. *Am J Pathol.* 2005, 166(2):565-573.

[91] Rafii S, Lyden D. Therapeutic stem and progenitor cell transplantation for organ vascularization and regeneration. *Nat Med* 2003(9):702-712.
[92] Rafii S, Avecilla S, Shmelkov S, Shido K, Tejada R, Moore MA, Heissig B, Hattori K. Angiogenic factors reconstitute hematopoiesis by recruiting stem cells from bone marrow microenvironment. *Ann N Y Acad Sci.* 2003, 996:49-60.
[93] Edelberg JM, Tang L, Hattori K, Lyden D, Rafii S. *Young adult bone marrow-derived endothelial precursor cells restore aging-impaired cardiac angiogenic function.* 2002, 90(10):E89-93.
[94] Quirici N, Soligo D, Caneva L, Servida F, Bossolasco P, Deliliers GL. Differentiation and expansion of endothelial cells from human bone marrow CD133(+) cells. *Br J Haematol.* 2001, 115(1):186-194.
[95] Baudouin S, Gillespie J, Anderson J, Dickinson A. A comparison of CFU-GM, BFU-E and endothelial progenitor cells using ex vivo expansion of selected cord blood CD133(+) and CD34(+) cells. *Cytotherapy.* 2007, 9(3):292-300.
[96] Fang N, Xie S, Wang S, Gao H, Wu C, Pan L. Construction of tissue engineered heart valves by using decellularized scaffolds and endothelial progenitor cells. *Chin Med J* 2007, 120(8):696-702.
[97] Ghajar CM, Blevins KS, Hughes CC, George SC, Putnam AJ. Mesenchymal stem cells enhance angiogenesis in mechanically viable prevascularized tissues via early matrix metalloproteinase upregulation. *Tissue Eng.* 2006, 12(10):2875-2888.
[98] Goussetis E, Manginas A, Koutelou M, Peristeri I, Theodosaki M, Kollaros N, Leontiadis E, Theodorakos A, Paterakis G, Karatasakis G, Cokkinos DV, Graphakos S. Intracoronary infusion of CD133+ and CD133-CD34+ selected autologous bone marrow progenitor cells in patients with chronic ischemic cardiomyopathy: cell isolation, adherence to the infarcted area, and body distribution. *Stem Cells.* 2006, 24(10):2279-2283.
[99] Reynolds BA, Weiss S. Generation of neurons and astrocytes from isolated cells of the adult mammalian central nervous system. *Science.* 1992;255(5052):1707-1710.
[100] Uchida N, Buck DW, He D, Reitsma MJ, Masek M, Phan TV, Tsukamoto AS, Gage, Weissman IL. Direct isolation of human central nervous system stem cells. *Proc Natl Acad Sci USA* 2000 97(26):14720-14725.

[101] Lois C., Alvarez-Buylla, A. Proliferating subventricular zone cells in the adult mammalian forebrain can differentiate into neurons and glia. *Proc. Natl Acad. Sci USA.*, 1993 90, 2074-2077.
[102] Reynolds BA, Weiss S. Generation of neurons and astrocytes from isolated cells of the adult mammalian central nervous system. *Science.* 1992, 27;255(5052):1707-1710.
[103] Gage F. H. Mammalian neural stem cells. *Science* 2000, 287:1433-1438.
[104] McKay R. Stem cells in the central nervous system. *Science* 1997, 276:66-71.
[105] Prajerova I, Honsa P, Chvatal A, Anderova M. Neural stem/progenitor cells derived from the embryonic dorsal telencephalon of D6/GFP mice differentiate primarily into neurons after transplantation into a cortical lesion. Cell Mol Neurobiol. 2009 *Cell Mol Neurobiol.* 2010;30(2):199-218.
[106] 1Kelly S, Bliss TM, Shah AK, Sun, Ma M, Foo WC, Masel J, Yenari MA, Weissman IL, Uchida N, Palmer T, Steinberg GK. Transplanted human fetal neural stem cells survive, migrate, and differentiate in ischemic rat cerebral cortex. *Proc Natl AcadSci U S A.* 2004;101(32):11839-11844.
[107] Tamaki SJ, Jacobs Y, Dohse M, Capela A, Cooper JD, Reitsma M, He D, Tushinski R, Belichenko PV, Salehi A, Mobley W, Gage, Huhn S, Tsukamoto AS, Weissman IL, Uchida N. Neuroprotection of host cells by human central nervous system stem cells in a mouse model of infantile neuronal ceroid lipofuscinosis. *Cell Stem Cell.* 2009;5(3):310-319.
[108] Lyly A, von Schantz C, Heine C, Schmiedt ML, Sipilä T, Jalanko A, Kyttälä A. Novel interactions of CLN5 support molecular networking between Neuronal Ceroid Lipofuscinosis proteins. *BMC Cell Biol.* 2009;10:83.
[109] Lyly A, von Schantz C, Salonen T, Kopra O, Saarela J, Jauhiainen M, Kyttälä A, Jalanko A. Glycosylation, transport, and complex formation of palmitoyl protein thioesterase 1 (PPT1)--distinct characteristics in neurons. *BMC Cell Biol.* 2007;12;8:22.
[110] Taupin P. HuCNS-SC (StemCells). *Curr Opin Mol Ther.* 2006;8(2):156-163.
[111] *www.stemcellsinc.com/news*

[91] Rafii S, Lyden D. Therapeutic stem and progenitor cell transplantation for organ vascularization and regeneration. *Nat Med* 2003(9):702-712.
[92] Rafii S, Avecilla S, Shmelkov S, Shido K, Tejada R, Moore MA, Heissig B, Hattori K. Angiogenic factors reconstitute hematopoiesis by recruiting stem cells from bone marrow microenvironment. *Ann N Y Acad Sci.* 2003, 996:49-60.
[93] Edelberg JM, Tang L, Hattori K, Lyden D, Rafii S. *Young adult bone marrow-derived endothelial precursor cells restore aging-impaired cardiac angiogenic function.* 2002, 90(10):E89-93.
[94] Quirici N, Soligo D, Caneva L, Servida F, Bossolasco P, Deliliers GL. Differentiation and expansion of endothelial cells from human bone marrow CD133(+) cells. *Br J Haematol.* 2001, 115(1):186-194.
[95] Baudouin S, Gillespie J, Anderson J, Dickinson A. A comparison of CFU-GM, BFU-E and endothelial progenitor cells using ex vivo expansion of selected cord blood CD133(+) and CD34(+) cells. *Cytotherapy*. 2007, 9(3):292-300.
[96] Fang N, Xie S, Wang S, Gao H, Wu C, Pan L. Construction of tissue engineered heart valves by using decellularized scaffolds and endothelial progenitor cells. *Chin Med J* 2007, 120(8):696-702.
[97] Ghajar CM, Blevins KS, Hughes CC, George SC, Putnam AJ. Mesenchymal stem cells enhance angiogenesis in mechanically viable prevascularized tissues via early matrix metalloproteinase upregulation. *Tissue Eng.* 2006, 12(10):2875-2888.
[98] Goussetis E, Manginas A, Koutelou M, Peristeri I, Theodosaki M, Kollaros N, Leontiadis E, Theodorakos A, Paterakis G, Karatasakis G, Cokkinos DV, Graphakos S. Intracoronary infusion of CD133+ and CD133-CD34+ selected autologous bone marrow progenitor cells in patients with chronic ischemic cardiomyopathy: cell isolation, adherence to the infarcted area, and body distribution. *Stem Cells.* 2006, 24(10):2279-2283.
[99] Reynolds BA, Weiss S. Generation of neurons and astrocytes from isolated cells of the adult mammalian central nervous system. *Science*. 1992;255(5052):1707-1710.
[100] Uchida N, Buck DW, He D, Reitsma MJ, Masek M, Phan TV, Tsukamoto AS, Gage, Weissman IL. Direct isolation of human central nervous system stem cells. *Proc Natl Acad Sci USA* 2000 97(26):14720-14725.

[101] Lois C., Alvarez-Buylla, A. Proliferating subventricular zone cells in the adult mammalian forebrain can differentiate into neurons and glia. *Proc. Natl Acad. Sci USA.*, 1993 90, 2074-2077.

[102] Reynolds BA, Weiss S. Generation of neurons and astrocytes from isolated cells of the adult mammalian central nervous system. *Science.* 1992, 27;255(5052):1707-1710.

[103] Gage F. H. Mammalian neural stem cells. *Science* 2000, 287:1433-1438.

[104] McKay R. Stem cells in the central nervous system. *Science* 1997, 276:66-71.

[105] Prajerova I, Honsa P, Chvatal A, Anderova M. Neural stem/progenitor cells derived from the embryonic dorsal telencephalon of D6/GFP mice differentiate primarily into neurons after transplantation into a cortical lesion. Cell Mol Neurobiol. 2009 *Cell Mol Neurobiol.* 2010;30(2):199-218.

[106] 1Kelly S, Bliss TM, Shah AK, Sun, Ma M, Foo WC, Masel J, Yenari MA, Weissman IL, Uchida N, Palmer T, Steinberg GK. Transplanted human fetal neural stem cells survive, migrate, and differentiate in ischemic rat cerebral cortex. *Proc Natl AcadSci U S A.* 2004;101(32):11839-11844.

[107] Tamaki SJ, Jacobs Y, Dohse M, Capela A, Cooper JD, Reitsma M, He D, Tushinski R, Belichenko PV, Salehi A, Mobley W, Gage, Huhn S, Tsukamoto AS, Weissman IL, Uchida N. Neuroprotection of host cells by human central nervous system stem cells in a mouse model of infantile neuronal ceroid lipofuscinosis. *Cell Stem Cell.* 2009;5(3):310-319.

[108] Lyly A, von Schantz C, Heine C, Schmiedt ML, Sipilä T, Jalanko A, Kyttälä A. Novel interactions of CLN5 support molecular networking between Neuronal Ceroid Lipofuscinosis proteins. *BMC Cell Biol.* 2009;10:83.

[109] Lyly A, von Schantz C, Salonen T, Kopra O, Saarela J, Jauhiainen M, Kyttälä A, Jalanko A. Glycosylation, transport, and complex formation of palmitoyl protein thioesterase 1 (PPT1)--distinct characteristics in neurons. *BMC Cell Biol.* 2007;12;8:22.

[110] Taupin P. HuCNS-SC (StemCells). *Curr Opin Mol Ther.* 2006;8(2):156-163.

[111] *www.stemcellsinc.com/news*

[112] Temeltas G, Dagci T, Kurt F, Evren V, Tuglu I. Bladder function recovery in rats with traumatic spinal cord injury after transplantation of neuronal-glial restricted precursors or bone marrow stromal cells. *J Urol.* 2009;181(6):2774-2779.
[113] Evans MJ, Kaufman MH. Establishment in culture of pluripotential cells from mouse embryos. *Nature* 1981;292:154-156.
[114] Martin GR. Isolation of a pluripotent cell line from early mouse embryos cultured in medium conditioned by teratocarcinoma stem cells. *PNAS U S A.* 1981;78(12): 7634–7638.
[115] Andrews PW. From teratocarcinomas to embryonic stem cells. *Philos Trans R Soc Lond B Biol Sci.* 2002; 357(1420): 405–417.
[116] Thomson JA, Itskovitz-Eldor J, Shapiro SS, Waknitz MA, Swiergiel JJ, Marshall VS, Jones JM. Embryonic stem cell lines derived from human blastocysts. *Science.* 1998;282(5391):1145-1147.
[117] Lerou PH, Daley GQ. Therapeutic potential of embryonic stem cells. *Blood Rev.* 2005;19(6):321-331.
[118] Henson JD, Reddel RR. Assaying and investigating alternative lengthening of telomeres activity in human cells and cancers. *FEBS Lett.* 2010 Jun 11.
[119] 1Chen G, Hou Z, Gulbranson DR, Thomson JA. Actin-myosin contractility is responsible for the reduced viability of dissociated human embryonic stem cells. *Cell Stem Cell.* 2010;7(2):240-248.
[120] Tulpule A, Lensch MW, Miller JD, Austin K, D'Andrea A, Schlaeger TM, Shimamura A, Daley GQ. Knockdown of Fanconi anemia genes in human embryonic stem cells reveals early developmental defects in the hematopoietic lineage. *Blood.* 2010;115(17):3453-3462.
[121] McKinney-Freeman SL, Naveiras O, Daley GQ. Isolation of hematopoietic stem cells from mouse embryonic stem cells. *Curr Protoc Stem Cell Biol.* 2008; Chapter 1:Unit 1F.3.
[122] Lu B, Malcuit C, Wang S, Girman S, Francis P, Lemieux L, Lanza R, Lund R. Long-term safety and function of RPE from human embryonic stem cells in preclinical models of macular degeneration. *Stem Cells.* 2009;27(9):2126-2135.
[123] Lu SJ, Li F, Vida L, Honig GR. CD34+CD38- hematopoietic precursors derived from human embryonic stem cells exhibit an embryonic gene expression pattern. *Blood.* 2004;103(11):4134-4141.
[124] Paige SL, Osugi T, Afanasiev OK, Pabon L, Reinecke H, Murry CE. Endogenous Wnt/beta-catenin signaling is required for cardiac differentiation in human embryonic stem cells. *PLoS One.* 2010;5(6):e11134.

[125] Annas GJ, Caplan A, Elias S. Stem cell politics, ethics and medical progress. *Nat Med.* 1999 ;5(12):1339-1341.
[126] Annas GJ. Ulysses and the fate of frozen embryos--reproduction, research, or destruction? *N Engl J Med.* 2000;343(5):373-376.
[127] Annas GJ, Elias S. Politics, morals and embryos. *Nature.* 2004;431(7004):19-20.
[128] Klimanskaya I, Chung Y, Becker S, Lu SJ, Lanza R. Human embryonic stem cell lines derived from single blastomeres. *Nature.* 2006;444(7118):481-485.
[129] Chung Y, Klimanskaya I, Becker S, Li T, Maserati M, Lu SJ, Zdravkovic T, Ilic D, Genbacev O, Fisher S, Krtolica A, Lanza R. Human embryonic stem cell lines generated without embryo destruction. *Cell Stem Cell.* 2008;2(2):113-117.
[130] Swijnenburg RJ, Schrepfer S, Govaert JA, Cao F, Ransohoff K, Sheikh AY, Haddad M, Connolly AJ, Davis MM, Robbins RC, Wu JC. Immunosuppressive therapy mitigates immunological rejection of human embryonic stem cell xenografts. *Proc Natl Acad Sci U S A.* 2008;105(35):12991-12996.
[131] Oottamasathien S, Wang Y, Williams K, Franco OE, Wills ML, Thomas JC, Saba K, Sharif-Afshar AR, Makari JH, Bhowmick NA, DeMarco RT, Hipkens S, Magnuson M, Brock JW 3rd, Hayward SW, Pope JC 4th, Matusik RJ. Directed differentiation of embryonic stem cells into bladder tissue. *Dev Biol.* 2007;304(2):556-566
[132] Thomas JC, Oottamasathien S, Makari JH, Honea L, Sharif-Afshar AR, Wang Y, Adams C, Wills ML, Bhowmick NA, Adams MC, Brock JW 3rd, Hayward SW, Matusik RJ, Pope JC 4th. Temporal-spatial protein expression in bladder tissue derived from embryonic stem cells. *J Urol.* 2008;180(4 Suppl):1784-1789.
[133] Frimberger D, Morales N, Gearhart JD, Gearhart JP, Lakshmanan Y. Human embryoid body-derived stem cells in tissue engineering-enhanced migration in co-culture with bladder smooth muscle and urothelium. *Urology.* 2006;67(6):1298-1303.
[134] Frimberger D, Morales N, Shamblott M, Gearhart JD, Gearhart JP, Lakshmanan Y. Human embryoid body-derived stem cells in bladder regeneration using rodent model. *Urology.* 2005 Apr;65(4):827-832.
[135] Shamblott MJ, Axelman J, Littlefield JW, Blumenthal PD, Huggins GR, Cui Y, Cheng L, Gearhart JD. Human embryonic germ cell derivatives express a broad range of developmentally distinct markers and proliferate extensively in vitro. *Proc Natl Acad Sci U S A.* 2001;98(1):113-118.

[136] Takahashi K, Yamanaka S. Induction of pluripotent stem cells from mouse embryonic and adult fibroblast cultures by defined factors. *Cell.* 2006;126(4):663-76.

[137] Takahashi K, Tanabe K, Ohnuki M, Narita M, Ichisaka T, Tomoda K, Yamanaka S. Induction of pluripotent stem cells from adult human fibroblasts by defined factors. *Cell.* 2007;131(5):861-872.

[138] Yu J, Vodyanik MA, Smuga-Otto K, Antosiewicz-Bourget J, Frane JL, Tian S, Nie J, Jonsdottir GA, Ruotti V, Stewart R, Slukvin II, Thomson JA. Induced pluripotent stem cell lines derived from human somatic cells. *Science.* 2007;318(5858):1917-1920.

[139] Moretti A, Bellin M, Welling A, Jung CB, Lam JT, Bott-Flügel L, Dorn T, Goedel A, Höhnke C, Hofmann F, Seyfarth M, Sinnecker D, Schömig A, Laugwitz KL. Patient-specific induced pluripotent stem-cell models for long-QT syndrome. *N Engl J Med.* 2010 Jul 21. [Epub ahead of print]

[140] Tsuji O, Miura K, Okada Y, Fujiyoshi K, Mukaino M, Nagoshi N, Kitamura K, Kumagai G, Nishino M, Tomisato S, Higashi H, Nagai T, Katoh H, Kohda K, Matsuzaki Y, Yuzaki M, Ikeda E, Toyama Y, Nakamura M, Yamanaka S, Okano H. Therapeutic potential of appropriately evaluated safe-induced pluripotent stem cells for spinal cord injury.*Proc Natl Acad Sci U S A.* 2010;107(28):12704-12709.

[141] Hu BY, Weick JP, Yu J, Ma LX, Zhang XQ, Thomson JA, Zhang SC. Neural differentiation of human induced pluripotent stem cells follows developmental principles but with variable potency. *Proc Natl Acad Sci U S A.* 2010;107(9):4335-4340.

[142] Alipio Z, Liao W, Roemer EJ, Waner M, Fink LM, Ward DC, Ma Y. Reversal of hyperglycemia in diabetic mouse models using induced-pluripotent stem (iPS)-derived pancreatic beta-like cells. *Proc Natl Acad Sci U S A.* 2010;107(30):13426-13431.

[143] Carette JE, Pruszak J, Varadarajan M, Blomen VA, Gokhale S, Camargo FD, Wernig M, Jaenisch R, Brummelkamp TR. Generation of iPSCs from cultured human malignant cells. *Blood.* 2010; 115(20):4039-4042.

[144] Ebert AD, Yu J, Rose FF Jr, Mattis VB, Lorson CL, Thomson JA, Svendsen CN. Induced pluripotent stem cells from a spinal muscular atrophy patient. *Nature.* 2009;457(7227):277-280.

[145] Dimos JT, Rodolfa KT, Niakan KK, Weisenthal LM, Mitsumoto H, Chung W, Croft GF, Saphier G, Leibel R, Goland R, Wichterle H, Henderson CE, Eggan K. Induced pluripotent stem cells generated

from patients with ALS can be differentiated into motor neurons. *Science.* 2008;321(5893):1218-1221.
[146] Staerk J, Dawlaty MM, Gao Q, Maetzel D, Hanna J, Sommer CA, Mostoslavsky G, Jaenisch R. Reprogramming of human peripheral blood cells to induced pluripotent stem cells. *Cell Stem Cell.* 2010;7(1):20-24.
[147] Kropp BP, Eppley BL, Prevel CD, Rippy MK, Harruff RC, Badylak SF, Adams MC, Rink RC, Keating MA. Experimental assessment of small intestinal submucosa as a bladder wall substitute. *Urology* 1995, 46(3):396-400.
[148] Merguerian PA, Reddy PP, Barrieras DJ, Wilson GJ, Woodhouse K, Bagli DJ, McLorie GA, Khoury AE. Acellular bladder matrix allografts in the regeneration of functional bladders: evaluation of large-segment (> 24 cm) substitution in a porcine model. *BJU Int* 2000, 85(7):894-898.
[149] Piechota HJ, Dahms SE, Nunes LS, Dahiya R, Lue TF, Tanagho EA. In vitro functional properties of the rat bladder regenerated by the bladder acellular matrix graft. *Journal of Urology* 1998, 159(5):1717-1724.
[150] Behravesh E, Yasko AW, Engel PS, Mikos AG. Synthetic Biodegradable Polymers for Orthopaedic Applications. *Clin Ortho Rel Res* 1999, 1 (367S):118-129.
[151] Yang J, Webb AR, Pickerill SJ, Hageman G, Ameer GA. Synthesis and evaluation of poly(diol citrate) biodegradable elastomers. *Biomaterials.* 2006, 27(9):1889-1898.
[152] Yang J, Motlagh D, Webb AR, Ameer GA. Novel biphasic elastomeric scaffold for small-diameter blood vessel tissue engineering. Tissue Eng. 2005, 11(11-12):1876-1886.
[153] Kang Y, Yang J, Khan S, Anissian L, Ameer GA. A new biodegradable polyester elastomer for cartilage tissue engineering. *J Biomed Mater Res A.* 2006, 77(2):331-9
[154] Engler AJ, Sen S, Sweeney HL, Discher DE. Matrix elasticity directs stem cell lineage specification. *Cell* 2006, 126(4):677-689.
[155] Rajangam K, Behanna HA, Hui MJ, Han X, Hulvat JF, Lomasney JW, Stupp SI. Heparin binding nanostructures to promote growth of blood vessels. *Nano Lett.* 2006 6(9):2086-2090.
[156] Edelman ER, Nugent MA, Karnovsky MJ. Perivascular and intravenous administration of basic fibroblast growth factor: vascular and solid organ deposition. *PNAS USA* 1993, 90:1513-1517.

[157] Chen, RR, Mooney DJ. Polymeric growth factor delivery strategies for tissue engineering. *Pharm Res* 2003, 20(8):1103-1112.
[158] Lazarous D, Shou M, Scheinowitz M, Hodge E, Thirumurti V, Kitsiou A, Stiber J, Lobo A, Hunsberger S, Guetta E, Epstein S, Unger E. Comparative effects of basic fibroblast growth factor and vascular endothelial growth factor on coronary collateral development and the arterial response to injury. *Circulation* 1996, 94:1074-1082.
[159] Murphy WL, Peters MC, Kohn DH, Mooney DJ. Sustained release of vascular endothelial growth factor from mineralized poly(lactide-co-glycolide) scaffolds for tissue engineering. *Biomaterials* 2000, 21(24):2521-2527.
[160] Kimura Y, Ozeki M, Inamoto T, Tabata Y. Time course of de novo adipogenesis in matrigel by gelatin microspheres incorporating basic fibroblast growth factor. *Tiss Eng* 2002, 8(4):603-613.
[161] Zhang, S. Fabrication of novel biomaterials through molecular self-assembly. Nat Biot 2003, 21(10):1171-1178.
[162] Kisiday J, Jin M, Kurz B, Hung H, Semino C, Zhang S, Grodzinsky AJ. Self-assembling peptide hydrogel fosters chondrocyte matrix production and cell division: implications for cartilage tissue repair. *PNAS USA* 2002, 99(15):9996-10001.
[163] Hartgerink JD, Beniash E, Stupp SI. Self-assembly and mineralization of peptide-amphiphile nanofibers. *Science* 2001, 294(5547):1684-1688.
[164] Hartgerink JD, Beniash E, Stupp SI. Peptide-amphiphile nanofibers: a versatile scaffold for the preparation of self-assembling materials. *PNAS USA* 2002, 99(8):5133-5138.
[165] Silva GA, Czeisler C, Niece KL, Beniash E, Harrington DA, Kessler JA, Stupp SI. Selective differentiation of neural progenitor cells by high-epitope density nanofibers. *Science* 2004, 303(5662):1352-1357.
[166] Keyt BA, Berleau LT, Nguyen HV, Chen H, Heinsohn H, Vandlen R, Ferrara N. The carboxyl terminal domain (111-165) of vascular endothelial growth factor is critical for its mitogenic potency. *J Biol Chem* 1996, 271(13):7788-7795.
[167] Cardin AD, Weintraub HJR. Molecular Modeling of Protein-Glycosaminoglycan Interactions. *Arteriosclerosis* 1989, 9(1):21-32.
[168] Kam L, Shain W, Turner JN, Bizios R. Axonal outgrowth of hippocampal neurons on micro-scale networks of polylysine-conjugated laminin. *Biomaterials*. 2001, 22(10):1049-1054.

[169] Kam L, Shain W, Turner JN, Bizios R. Selective adhesion of astrocytes to surfaces modified with immobilized peptides. *Biomaterials* 2002, 23(2):511-515.

[170] Matsuzawa M, Weight FF, Potember RS, Liesi P. Directional neurite outgrowth and axonal differentiation of embryonic hippocampal neurons are promoted by a neurite outgrowth domain of the B2-chain of laminin. *Int J Dev Neurosci.* 1996, 4(3):283-295.

[171] Wei YT, Tian WM, Yu X, Cui FZ, Hou SP, Xu QY, Lee IS. Hyaluronic acid hydrogels with IKVAV peptides for tissue repair and axonal regeneration in an injured rat brain. *Biomed Mater.* 2007, 2(3):S142-S146.

[172] Tysseling-Mattiace VM, Sahni V, Niece KL, Birch D, Czeisler C, Fehlings MG, Stupp SI, Kessler JA. Self-assembling nanofibers inhibit glial scar formation and promote axon elongation after spinal cord injury. *J Neurosci.* 2008, 28(14):3814-3823.

[173] Nakamura M, Yamaguchi K, Mie M, Nakamura M, Akita K, Kobatake E. Promotion of angiogenesis by an artificial extracellular matrix protein containing the laminin-1-derived IKVAV sequence. *Bioconjug Chem. Bioconjug Chem.* 2009;20(9):1759-1764.

[174] Rivera FJ, Couillard-Despres S, Pedre X, Ploetz S, Caioni M, Lois C, Bogdahn U, Aigner L. Mesenchymal stem cells instruct oligodendrogenic fate decision on adult neural stem cells. *Stem Cells.* 2006, 24(10):2209-2219.

Index

A

aberrant cellular behavior, vii
acid, 5, 21, 29, 30, 37, 57
action potential, 22
AD, 46, 54, 56
adhesion, 57
adipose, 18, 45
adults, 43
adventitia, 2
age, 50, 51, 55
aggregation, 33
alanine, 39
allogenic cell sources, viii
ALS, 55
amino, 21, 37
amplitude, 22
anatomy, 1, 42
anemia, 52
angiogenesis, 16, 19, 31, 32, 50, 57
angiogenic process, 20
antibody, 21, 25
antithesis, 24
apex, 1
arthritis, 46
assessment, 55
astrocytes, 21, 39, 50, 51, 57

atherosclerotic plaque, 15
atrophy, 54
attachment, 32
autologous cell sources, vii, 24
autonomic nervous system, 2

B

base, 1
biodegradable matrices, viii
biological sciences, vii
biomaterials, 17, 33, 56
biomolecules, 35
biopsy, 5
bladder abnormalities, vii
bladder cancer, vii, 41
bladder tissue engineering, iv, vii, viii, 23
blood, 1, 6, 11, 19, 30, 47, 50, 55
blood vessels, 1, 6, 19, 30, 55
bonding, 33
bone, 9, 11, 13, 15, 17, 19, 23, 30, 31, 41, 44, 45, 46, 47, 48, 49, 50, 52
bone cells, 30
bone marrow, 9, 11, 13, 17, 19, 41, 44, 45, 46, 47, 48, 49, 50, 52

bone marrow transplant, 17, 18
bones, 11
bowel, 3
brain, 21, 57
by-products, 30

C

cancer, vii, 41
candidates, 28
carboxyl, 37, 56
carcinoma, 23
cardiomyopathy, 50
cardiovascular system, 49
cartilage, 15, 23, 30, 55, 56
cartilaginous, 30
cell biology, vii, 41, 42
cell culture, 23, 30
cell differentiation, 17, 24, 32, 39, 45, 46
cell division, 56
cell fusion, 47
cell line, 23, 41, 52, 53, 54, 55
cell surface, 18, 20
central nervous system(CNS), 21, 50, 51
cerebral cortex, 22, 51
children, 12, 44, 46
chondrocyte, 56
clinical bladder tissue engineering, vii
clinical problems, 3
clinical trials, 24
clusters, 23
CNS, 21
collagen, 7, 17, 33, 39, 45
collateral, 56
compatibility, 30
compliance, 3, 30, 43
complications, 3
composites, 7
composition, 7
compounds, 41
connective tissue, 1, 13
consensus, 37
constituents, 18
coordination, 22
copolymers, 29
cornea, 48
cortex, 22, 51
cortical neurons, 22
cryopreservation, 47
cues, 11
culture, 30, 44, 52, 53
cystectomy, vii
cystoplasty, 3, 42
cytokines, 13

D

damaged tissue, vii
defects, vii, 3, 11, 41, 52
deficiencies, 31
deficiency, 22
degradation, 30
deposition, 55
derivatives, 22, 53
destruction, 24, 53
developmental defects, 3, 11, 52
diffusion, 37
disease model, 22
diseases, 12, 46
distribution, 48, 50
donors, 17
drainage, 1
drug targets, 43
drug therapy, 43

E

ECM, 29, 37
ECs, 19
ectoderm, 23
education, 4
elasticity modulus, 30
elastomers, 39, 55
electrolyte, 3
elongation, 57
elucidation, 24
embryogenesis, 19
embryonic stem cells, 9, 24, 52, 53
endoderm, 23
endothelial cells, 13, 19, 48, 50
endothelial cells (ECs), 19
endothelium, 19, 37
engineering, iv, vii, viii, 5, 9, 19, 23, 32, 37, 41, 43, 44, 47, 53, 55, 56
enterocystoplasty, vii
environment, 9, 20, 22, 24, 31, 39
enzyme, 22, 23
EPC, 19
epithelial cells, 48
epithelium, 23
epitopes, 20, 41
ESCs, 41
ethics, 53
evidence, 13, 19, 25, 47, 48
exposure, 35
expulsion, 1
extracellular matrix, 39, 49, 57

F

Fabrication, 56
fat, 15
fertilization, 23
fibers, 1, 15, 33, 35, 49
fibrin, 20
fibroblast growth factor, 13, 44, 55, 56
fibroblasts, 9, 11, 23, 27, 54
films, 44
financial, 3
first generation, 27
fluid, 35
forebrain, 51
formation, 3, 17, 18, 20, 25, 29, 30, 39, 41, 51, 57
fusion, 16, 47, 49

G

GABA, 21
gel, 33, 35
gelation, 35
gene expression, 52
genes, 13, 15, 52
germ cells, 25
germ layer, 23, 27
glia, 51
glial cells, 21, 22
glycosaminoglycans, 29
growth, viii, 13, 20, 21, 23, 29, 30, 31, 32, 37, 39, 41, 44, 45, 46, 55, 56
growth factor, 13, 20, 21, 23, 29, 30, 32, 37, 41, 44, 45, 46, 55, 56

H

harvesting, 24, 30
healing, 19
health care, 3
heart valves, 19, 50
hematopoietic stem cells, 11, 52
hepatocytes, 47

host, 5, 11, 22, 24, 33, 51
human, 1, 3, 11, 13, 22, 23, 27, 42, 43, 44, 45, 46, 47, 49, 50, 51, 52, 53, 54, 55
hydrogels, 57
hydrogen, 33
hydrolysis, 29
hydronephrosis, 3
hydroxyapatite, 46
hyperglycemia, 54
hyperplasia, 16

I

ideal, 12, 22, 24
identification, 21, 23, 45
immune response, 24, 31
immunosuppressive therapies, 22
in vitro, 7, 13, 23, 44, 45, 46, 53
in vivo, 21, 24, 30, 35, 39, 45, 48
income, 4
individuals, 4
induction, 21, 24, 32
infarction, 21
infection, 3
inflammatory cells, 15, 24
inhibition, 14
injury, 3, 15, 18, 19, 22, 24, 47, 49, 52, 54, 56, 57
insertion, 27
integration, 15
integrin, 46
integrity, 19
interface, 11
internal mechanisms, 21
intervention, 3, 41
intestine, 3
islands, 19
isolation, 21, 23, 46, 50
isoleucine, 39

K

karyotype, 24
kidney, 48
kidneys, 1
kinetics, 14, 46, 47

L

lactic acid, 29
laws, 24
lead, 3, 21, 25
LFA, 13
lifetime, 3
liver, 19, 47
lumen, 1
Luo, 46
lymph node, 45
lymphocytes, 13
lysine, 39

M

macromolecules, 35
macrophages, 13
macular degeneration, 52
malignant cells, 54
management, 42
marrow, 9, 11, 12, 13, 17, 19, 41, 44, 45, 46, 47, 48, 49, 50, 52
Mars, 45
mass, 23, 25
materials, vii, 17, 25, 29, 41, 56, 57
materials science, vii, 41
matrix, 3, 18, 19, 29, 39, 45, 49, 50, 55, 56, 57
matrix metalloproteinase, 50
MB, 48
mechanical properties, 30

media, 13
Medicaid, 4
medical, 4, 53
medical care, 4
Medicare, 4
medicine, vii, 15, 19, 24, 25, 28
mesenchymal stem cells, 11, 18, 45, 46, 47
mesenchyme, 24
mesoderm, 23
metalloproteinase, 50
mice, 15, 17, 22, 45, 47, 51
microspheres, 56
migration, 19, 53
mineralization, 56
mitogen, 45
models, 6, 21, 27, 52, 54
modulus, 30
molecular weight, 29
molecules, 30, 33, 35, 37, 39
motor neurons, 55
MR, 45
mucosa, 1
mucus, 3
multipotent, 9, 15
murder, 24
muscle contraction, 2
muscles, 49
mutation, 22
myelomeningocele, vii, 7
myosin, 52

N

nanofibers, 35, 56, 57
nanomaterials, 22
nanostructures, 55
nanotechnology, 31, 32, 41
negative effects, 11
neovascularization, 19, 32, 48

nervous system, 2, 21, 50, 51
networking, 51
neural networks, 28
neurofilaments, 21
neurogenesis, 21
neurogenic bladder, vii, 2, 3, 4, 7, 8, 20, 42, 43, 44
neuronal cells, 39
neurons, 2, 21, 50, 51, 55, 56, 57
neuroprotection, 22
neurotransmitters, 21
nodes, 45
nutrients, 9, 23

O

organ, vii, 19, 25, 50, 55

P

pathophysiology, 43
pediatric urologists, vii
peptide, 31, 35, 39, 56
peptides, 57
perforation, 3
performers, 2
periosteum, 11
peripheral blood, 47, 55
peripheral nervous system, 21
pH, 33, 35
phenotype, 12, 16, 30, 32, 44, 46, 48, 49
phospholipids, 33
physical properties, 29
physiological function, vii, 2, 18, 22, 25, 28, 31, 41
physiology, 43
politics, 53
polycondensation, 30

polyesters, 30
polymer, 5, 29, 30
polysaccharide, 37
population, 4, 18, 19, 25, 31
precursor cells, 13, 17, 50
preparation, iv, 56
principles, vii, 54
progenitor cells, 9, 11, 14, 19, 21, 39, 46, 47, 48, 50, 51, 56
proliferation, 7, 19, 23, 29, 32
proteins, 1, 29, 32, 37, 39, 42, 51
proteoglycans, 29
pubis, 1

Q

quality of life, 4

R

radical cystectomy, vii
reactions, 30
reactivity, 21
receptors, 35
recognition, 35
recombination, 24
reconstruction, 3, 17, 44
recovery, 16, 52
recruiting, 31, 50
regenerate, 5
regeneration, 5, 8, 9, 12, 15, 17, 19, 25, 28, 29, 30, 31, 32, 39, 41, 44, 48, 49, 50, 53, 55, 57
regenerative medicine, 15, 19, 24, 25, 28
rejection, 24, 53
relaxation, 2, 42, 43
renal failure, 3
repair, 15, 17, 48, 56, 57

reproduction, 53
researchers, 27, 37
resection, vii
respiration, 29
response, 2, 17, 19, 24, 49, 56
restoration, vii, 32
routes, 28

S

safety, 22, 52
science, vii, 41
seeding, 30
self-assembly, 56
septic arthritis, 46
serum, 13
sham, 17, 18
signals, 15, 31
sinuses, 45
skeletal muscle, 15, 49
smooth muscle, 1, 2, 5, 6, 7, 9, 12, 16, 18, 20, 23, 25, 28, 30, 32, 42, 43, 44, 48, 49, 53
smooth muscle cells, 1, 5, 7, 9, 25, 42, 44, 48, 49
Social Security Administration, 4
societal cost, 4
solution, 33, 35
somatic cell, 27, 54
SP, 45, 47, 49, 57
special education, 4
species, 13
sphincter, 2, 3, 43
spina bifida, vii, 3, 11, 41, 42, 43
spinal cord, 21, 22, 24, 35, 43, 52, 54, 57
spinal cord injury, 22, 24, 52, 54, 57
spleen, 45
sprouting, 39
state, viii, 2, 7, 27, 46

states, 11, 27
stem cell biology, vii, 41
stem cell differentiation, 45
stem cell lines, 52, 53, 54
stem cells, 9, 11, 15, 17, 23, 27, 45, 46, 47, 48, 50, 51, 52, 53, 54, 55, 57
stimulation, 21, 46
storage, 1, 2, 3
stress, 4
striatum, 21
stroma, 11, 45
stromal cells, 45, 46, 49, 52
structural protein, 29, 37
submucosa, 5, 17, 44, 55
suboptimal bladder function, vii
substitution, 55
substrate, 30
substrates, 29
Sun, 51
surface area, 5
surgical intervention, 3, 41
suture, 30
syndrome, 43, 54
synergistic effect, vii, 20, 31
synovial fluid, 35
synthesis, 30, 45
synthetic polymers, vii, 29

T

T cell, 24
target, vii, 15, 31
techniques, 8, 24, 30, 41
technology, 5, 39
telencephalon, 51
testing, 21
TGF, 29, 32
therapy, 43, 53
thin films, 44

thymus, 45
tissue, iv, vii, viii, 1, 5, 6, 7, 9, 11, 13, 15, 19, 21, 23, 24, 27, 29, 30, 31, 32, 37, 39, 41, 44, 50, 53, 55, 56, 57
tissue engineering, iv, vii, viii, 5, 9, 19, 23, 32, 37, 41, 44, 53, 55, 56
trafficking, 49
traits, 27
transcription factors, 27
transformation, 27
transforming growth factor, 46
transgene, 45
transplant, 18, 21
transplantation, 18, 21, 33, 49, 50, 51, 52
transport, 51
transurethral resection, vii
trauma, vii, 41
treatment, vii, 3, 5, 7, 20, 30, 44
trial, 7, 22
turnover, 48

U

umbilical cord, 47
uniform, 29, 30
United States, vii
ureters, 1
urethra, 1, 42
urinary bladder, iv, 1, 17, 44, 49
urinary tract, 3, 17, 42, 43
urinary tract infection, 3
urine, 1, 3
urothelium, 1, 6, 25, 53
USA, 50, 51, 55, 56

V

vagina, 1
valine, 39
valuation, 30
vascularization, 31, 41, 50
vasculature, 9, 20, 28, 30, 41, 49
vehicles, 41
vein, 16, 49
vesicle, 1
vessels, 1, 6, 19, 30, 45, 55
voiding, 2, 22

W

water, 1
wild type, 18
wound healing, 19

X

xenografts, 53

Y

yolk, 19